An Introduction to the Profession of Medical Technology

THIRD EDITION

M. RUTH WILLIAMS, Ph.D., MT (ASCP)

Professor Emeritus
Department of Medical Technology
College of Health Related Professions
University of Florida, Gainesville

DAVID S. LINDBERG, Ed.D., MT (ASCP)

Associate Dean and Associate Professor
of Medical Technology

Louisiana State University Medical Center
School of Allied Health Professions

New Orleans, Louisiana

Lea & Febiger   1979   Philadelphia

Library of Congress Cataloging in Publication Data

Williams, Margaret Ruth.

  An introduction to the profession of medical technology.

  Includes index.

  1. Medical technology—Vocational guidance.
I. Lindberg, David S., joint author.   II. Title.

RB37.6.W55   1979   610.69'53   79-672

ISBN 0-8121-0667-9

1st Edition, 1971
    Reprinted, 1973
2nd Edition, 1975
    Reprinted, 1977
3rd Edition, 1979

Published in Great Britain by
Henry Kimpton Publishers, London

PRINTED IN THE UNITED STATES OF AMERICA

Foreword to the First Edition

Medical technology in the past decade has grown from a health occupation to a health profession. As medical technologists have developed more of their own body of knowledge and as they have questioned more of their techniques and procedures in the laboratory, they have become true health professionals. The tasks of medical technologists and other allied health personnel in the laboratory will require highly competent and superbly educated persons performing more and more complicated scientific processes.

The medical technologist of tomorrow will have to assume responsibilities and perform duties that no one has thought of today. Medical technologists are moving to become managers of doers rather than doers. They will perform roles of supervisors, teachers, and administrators. The roles they previously assumed will be performed by those with post-high school and junior college education working under the direction and supervision of the medical technologist. The medical technologist of tomorrow will in reality become the clinical pathologist's assistant.

The technological advances that took us to the moon will take us to new heights in the delivery of health care. The medical laboratory of today does not resemble one of only a few years ago, and as in all of society, the most constant factor is change. Students in medical technology will require much more preparation in biophysics, bioenvironmental medicine, and basic electronics. The curricula for medical technologists, medical laboratory technicians, and certified laboratory assistants must be continually revised to meet the needs of tomorrow for laboratory personnel in the allied health occupations and professions.

The author of this most needed text is well qualified for the assignment. She joined the staff of the College of Health Related Professions in 1961 as Head of the Department of Medical Technology. She had been a medical technologist for twenty-eight years previous to this assignment. She has served on the Board of Schools, a standing committee of the American Society of Clinical Pathologists, for a four year term. She was a member of the Joint Committee of the American Association of Junior Colleges and the National Committee on Medical Technology Education for three years. Since 1965 she has been on the editorial staff of the *American Journal of Medical Technology,* and she is the author of numerous articles.

It is indeed heartening that this medical technologist, educator, and administrator should share her experience and knowledge with the many university, college, and junior college students who will be preparing for careers in medical technology. This book will also be found useful in counseling high school students seeking career information.

DARREL J. MASE, DEAN EMERITUS
College of Health Related Professions
University of Florida
Gainesville, Florida

Preface to the Second Edition

This book is the direct outgrowth of requests from students for a textbook in an introductory course in medical technology. Although it is intended primarily as a textbook, guidance counselors should find it a useful tool in counseling high school or junior college students. Medical technologists may find it of interest as a reference on the historical background of the profession.

Insofar as possible, information concerning the development of medical technology has been obtained from the bylaws and reports published by the American Society of Clinical Pathologists, reports and bylaws of the American Society for Medical Technology, and "A Short History of the Registry of Medical Technologists," the presidential address of Dr. Lall Montgomery at the 1967 convention of the American Society of Clinical Pathologists. Dr. Montgomery was the second chairman of the Board of Registry, holding this position from 1940 to 1964.

The second edition has been enlarged in several areas and completely updated. However, even the most dedicated effort to reflect the current status fails because of the rapid progress in the profession.

It is a pleasure to welcome a co-author, Dr. David Lindberg. Dr. Lindberg is well known in medical technology, particularly for his contributions in the field of education. There is no doubt that subsequent editions will incorporate some of the same enthusiasm and vitality he demonstrates as a professional educator.

I wish to thank the host of people who encouraged me to write this book. Special thanks are extended to the Registry of Medical Technologists, American Society of Clinical Pathologists; Dr. Lall Montgomery; Mrs. Ruth Drummond; the executive office of the American Society for Medical Technology; and my colleagues at the University of Florida.

Gainesville, Florida   M. RUTH WILLIAMS

Preface to the Third Edition

This third edition required numerous revisions to update information about credentialing, professional societies, and many other facets of our profession. We found the revision process to be highly interesting yet frustrating, as the source materials were assembled and organized, and as the patterns of change that have taken place during the past four years began to be apparent. We were forcefully reminded that the clinical laboratory professions are just as dynamic in their constant change as are the technologies employed by clinical laboratory professionals. The process was frustrating since more changes will occur before the edition can be published.

The many references and explanations of historical background have been retained from previous editions, so that the interested reader may have the opportunity to perceive just how much change has taken place in the professions in such a short period of years.

We are indebted to many persons who have assisted in the preparation of this edition through providing information, reviewing manuscript drafts, and who submitted helpful suggestions and comments to the publishers. Special thanks go to Sara Marie Cicarelli, Chester Dziekonski, and Lynn Silver, who supplied information and assistance concerning their respective agencies and organizations.

A sincere thank you is extended to Lea & Febiger for their continued interest, cooperation and encouragement.

Gainesville, Florida   M. Ruth Williams
New Orleans, Louisiana   David S. Lindberg

Contents

1

A Definition of Medical Technology

Many definitions have been proposed for the term, medical technology. Heinemann,[1] a medical technologist, defined it as "the application of principles of natural, physical, and biological sciences to the performance of laboratory procedures which aid in the diagnosis and treatment of disease." The definition by Fagelson,[2] also a medical technologist, is perhaps preferable, since it adds an important dimension. She considers medical technology to be "that branch of medicine concerned with the performance of the laboratory determinations and analyses used in the diagnosis and treatment of disease and the *maintenance of health.*" These laboratory determinations and analyses are performed in the clinical laboratory by the medical technologist, a person who has obtained a sound foundation in the scientific principles involved and a proficiency in the performance of the test procedures. Detailed information on professional preparation will be found in Chapter 5.

The director of the clinical laboratory usually is a pathologist. A pathologist is, first of all, a physician, either a doctor of medicine or a doctor of osteopathy. His specialty is pathology, which is defined by the American Board of Pathology as "that specialty of the practice of medicine which contributes to diagnosis, prognosis and treatment through knowledge gained by laboratory applications of the biologic, chemical or physical sciences to man, or material obtained from man."[3] Pathology is further divided into two areas—anatomic and clinical. The physician preparing to be a pathologist may elect to specialize in either anatomic pathology or clinical pathology or both. If he is interested in the diagnosis or confirmation of diseases through autopsy examination and cellular differentiation of autopsy and surgical tissues, he may wish to specialize in anatomic pathology only. If he is more interested in the chemical, microbiological (study of bacteria), and hematological (study of blood) procedures, he may decide to specialize in clinical pathology.

In order to be eligible for certification by the American Board of Pathology in both clinical and anatomic pathology, the candidate must have taken four years of "combined training" in an institution approved by the Liaison Committee on Graduate Medical Education of the American Medical Association, or by the Board.[4] The time is equally divided between the two areas. In addition to the residency, he must have one more year of training, either an internship or further study in pathology.

"Combined training" may be defined as a total of four years of training in at least two of five subspecialty areas. Successful passing of an examination in the specialty in which certification is desired gives the candidate board certification, or in the vernacular, he has his "Boards."

In the Final Report of the Commission on Medical Education (1932)[5] is found this statement:

> The more scientific laboratory determinations become, and the wider the field of their application, the more thoroughly trained must the physician be to interpret, correlate, and utilize the findings of the laboratory in relation to the problem of the individual patient.

The years since this report have seen a marked increase in the variety of laboratory procedures available. New procedures are added as new knowledge and equipment make them possible. The extreme complexity of these procedures often makes it necessary for the physician to rely on the pathologist for assistance. The pathologist performs the role of interpreting and correlating for the physician the results obtained by the medical technologist in order that the physician may use them in the diagnosis and treatment of the patient. Thus, the pathologist and the medical technologist work together with the physician as members of a team whose goal at all times is better patient care.

The title of this book indicates a rather firm conviction that medical

2

technology is a profession. Perhaps it would be appropriate to quote from a publication of the American Society for Medical Technology.[6]

Becoming a profession is a gradual process. There are basic qualifications that must be met to be an accepted, established profession. Because the profession of medical technology is in the process of fulfilling these qualifications, it is classified as an emerging profession. This presents many challenges to technologists individually and collectively. To fulfill the requirements of a profession members must jointly strive to:

a. Acquire differential technological expertise
b. Establish and maintain standards of excellence
c. Formulate a code of ethics
d. Establish and enforce rules of conduct
e. Establish and enforce minimum qualifications for entrance into the profession
f. Allow opportunities for human service
g. Set criteria for recruitment and training
h. Develop a sense of responsibility to the profession, to colleagues and to society as a whole
i. Insure a measure of protection for members
j. Establish collective control
k. Endeavor to elevate their profession to a position of dignity and social standing in society
l. Organize and develop a professional, qualifying association

Medical technology, as will be seen in subsequent chapters, does not meet several of these criteria. Since these criteria are similar to those qualifications usually attributed to professions, honesty compels the author to agree that medical technology can only be called an emerging profession.

REFERENCES

1. Heinemann, Ruth: What is medical technology? Hosp. Prog., *44*:96-98, 1963.
2. Fagelson, Anna: *Opportunities in Medical Technology.* New York, Vocational Guidance Manuals, Inc., 1961 (Out of print).
3. *Directory of Medical Specialists.* Vol. XIII. Chicago, Von Hoffman Press, 1968.
4. *Directory of Medical Specialists.* 18th Ed., 1. Chicago, Marquis Who's Who, 1977.
5. Commission on Medical Education: *Final Report of the Commission on Medical Education.* 1932.
6. *Personnel Relations Handbook.* Cadence 1, No. 2. Mar., 1970, p 19.

SUGGESTED READINGS

Heinemann, Ruth: What is medical technology? Hosp. Prog. *44:*96-98, 1963.

Anderson, Ellen: Medical technology today. Am. J. Med. Technol. *31:*159-168, 1965.

Key, Patricia: Medical technology, profession or skilled labor? A student's point of view. Am. J. Med. Technol. *31:*219-223, 1965.

White, Lavinia: Thirty-five years of medical technology. Am. J. Med. Technol. *31:*295-299, 1965.

2

A Brief History of Medical Technology

Where does one look for the beginning of a profession? Herrick,[1] a medical technologist, traces the beginning of medical technology back to 1500 B.C. when intestinal parasites such as taenia and ascaris were mentioned in writings. She also notes that in the *Ebers Papyrus* (a "recipe" book for treatment of diseases) there is a description of the three different stages of hookworm infection. Both taenia and ascaris are large parasites, very characteristic in appearance, and would require no specialized knowledge to identify. All three stages of hookworm produce small forms that would demand more sophisticated study. This identification of intestinal parasites is done today in the parasitology division of the clinical laboratory.

Probably the most commonly performed laboratory test today is the urinalysis. Examination of the urine dates back to antiquity. Early Hindu doctors made the "scientific" observation that the urine of certain individuals attracted ants, and that such urine had a sweetish taste. During the Medieval period (1096–1438) urinalysis was a fad. Quacks calling themselves doctors reaped fortunes from diagnosing diseases by the appearance of the urine. In most cases the correlation between the diagnosed disease and the condition of the patient must have been coincidental.

The writings of Hippocrates who lived from 460 to 370 B.C. indicate he had a knowledge of tuberculosis, malaria, mumps, anthrax,

5

and purpural septicemia (childbed fever). His observations, however, were clinical rather than pathologic.

Fagelson[2] prefers to date medical technology from the 14th century when a prominent Italian physician at the University of Bologna employed one Alessandra Giliani to perform certain tasks which would now be considered those of the technologist. It may be of interest that this young lady died from a laboratory acquired infection.

During the 16th century Ambroise Paré contributed materially to the advance of anatomy, pathology, medicine, and surgery. He made pathology popular in France through his many postmortem examinations. His examinations included at least three members of royalty—Henry II, the king of Navarre, and Charles IX.[3]

The 17th century saw the invention of the microscope. We often associate Leeuwenhoek (1632–1723) with this invention, but compound microscopes had already been developed prior to his work. However, he improved the lenses and was the first to describe red blood cells, to see protozoa, and to classify bacteria according to shape. With the invention of the microscope, microbiology and pathology progressed rapidly, yet the beginning of pathology is not clearly defined.

Malpighi (1628–1694) was described as the "greatest of the early microscopists and his work in embryology and anatomy definitely marks him as the founder of pathology."[1] Kracke,[4] Gauss,[3] and many others do not agree with this statement but believe that pathology as it is practiced dates only from the time of Virchow, making it one of the youngest of the medical specialties. "In the 19th century the cell theory was enunciated and established; pathology was placed on a cellular basis; chemistry witnessed the rapid discovery and isolation of numerous elements; organic chemistry came into existence to be followed rapidly by physiological chemistry which paved the way for the newer blood chemistry."[3] Laboratory tests were greatly improved, moving from qualitative to quantitative. In 1848 Fehling performed the first quantitative test for urine sugar.

Virchow (1821–1902) saw the beginning of the organized advancement of science. His interests, while mainly in cellular physiology, included anthropology and physiology, and his publications covered many fields. He founded the Archives of Pathology in Berlin in 1847.

With the production of aniline dyes about the middle of the 19th century it became possible to stain bacteria and to study them under the microscope. Concurrently, the rapid advancement in the knowledge of chemical compounds and reactions laid the groundwork for the development of our modern clinical chemistry.

6

THE FIRST LABORATORIES

Perhaps the first chemical laboratory related to medicine to be opened in this country was that at the University of Michigan. Dr. Victor V. Vaughan,[5] who later became dean of the University of Michigan College of Medicine, wrote:

> Dr. Douglas (not otherwise identified) began laboratory instruction on his appointment in 1844 and soon secured from the Regents a fund sufficient to erect a small one-story laboratory and in this the students were soon busy in a field hitherto unknown and unvisited by medical students in this country at least. This small laboratory, well equipped for the times, grew year by year until it soon became the largest and best equipped chemical laboratory open to students in this country.
>
> Nor was laboratory chemical teaching confined to medical students. Students in the collegiate department anticipating medicine or any other calling in which this science might be useful availed themselves of the opportunities.

This laboratory was not hospital connected, however. The medical school did not open until 1850, and no hospital facilities were available until 1875. The department of pathology was established at the same time as the medical school.

Dr. Vaughan worked as a laboratory assistant in 1874 during his medical training. He tells that he examined urines and blood "and later the stomach contents" of the patients who were being presented to the class. He does not clarify what he meant by "later." He wrote: "I remember with what pride I demonstrated leukemic blood and urine to the class; how I exhibited crystals of tyrosine and leucine in the urine in a case of cancer of the liver, a rare opportunity indeed; how I showed the presence of urea in the perspiration of a man dying of kidney disease."[5] Today, nearly a century later, we still do these tests, although we demonstrate leukemic blood and urea by more sophisticated methods. We still search for crystals of tyrosine and leucine and still find them but rarely.

Other hospitals were recognizing the need for pathologists. At the first meeting of the staff of Cook County Hospital in Chicago (1865) the position of pathologist and "curator of the dead house" was established.[6]

In 1878 Dr. William H. Welch, who had studied pathology and bacteriology in Germany, returned to this country to look for a position. Because of the fine reputation of the College of Physicians and Surgeons in New York and because it was his alma mater, he first applied there. This hospital had never had any laboratories, but he was told if he could find any room not otherwise assigned he could set up one. He found none. Denied a job there, he went to the Bellevue

Hospital Medical College. He finally obtained a laboratory which, he said, "I shall have for giving microscopal courses and for teaching." His laboratory consisted of three rooms furnished with kitchen tables. He was later quoted as saying the college spent "fully $25 in equipping the laboratory." Somehow he acquired six antique microscopes and started his first students. According to Flexner,[7] this was the first laboratory course in pathology ever given in an American medical school.

In 1885 Welch became the first professor of pathology at Johns Hopkins University.[8] Here he was assigned to a small two-story building remodeled according to his specifications. On the ground floor were the bacteriological laboratory and the two-story high amphitheater for autopsies. On the second floor was the pathological laboratory. Welch was given a budget of $2,000 which he promptly overspent. Items purchased included $393 for glassware and $26 for a refrigerator. The specialties taught were pathology, bacteriology, and experimental pathology. Since the hospital had not yet opened, it was necessary to find another source of clinical material. For several years the source was the Bay View Insane Asylum.

Several references in the literature indicate that the first clinical laboratory was opened in 1896. One of these states that this laboratory was at Johns Hopkins Hospital, that it occupied a room 12 × 12, and was equipped at a cost of $50.[9] Another source states, ". . . one of the earliest clinical pathology laboratories was set up in 1896 with equipment valued at $300 . . ."[2]

Camac's article[10] is probably the source of all the references made to size and cost of hospital laboratories, yet a careful study of the article raises the question whether the laboratories to which Camac referred were indeed the hospital laboratories. He indicates a clinical laboratory had been opened at the University of Pennsylvania in 1896 (William Pepper Laboratory) and that others were to be found in Boston, Baltimore, New York, "and in many other cities . . . all having sprung into life in the short space of about 20 years." His refutation to the objection that laboratories require space states: "The clinical laboratory, with its complicated chemical apparatus, spectroscope and polariscope, nitrogen-estimating apparatus, etc., does require space." He goes on to say that "Only the perfected and simplified methods and apparatus have place in the hospital and ward clinical laboratory. This apparatus and these methods are of such simple nature that they can be transported to the bedside. It does not, therefore, require much space to accommodate them. With the hearty cooperation of the authorities, the writer established such ward laboratories at Johns Hopkins Hospital in 1896, and at Bellevue Hospital in 1899. The area required for this ward laboratory is about 6 × 6 or 10 × 10 feet, a window being the only essential. Indeed, a window and a table are the only essentials in the matter of space. While running water and gas are helpful adjuncts, the ordinary water-bottle and spirit-lamp are all that is necessary. Probably no part of a hospital is more modest in its demands than the ward laboratory."

This, then, is the explanation for the descriptions of sizes of rooms, for one of the pictures accompanying the article has a picture of the ward laboratory, and lists the size of the room as 12 × 12. In our opinion, these laboratories cannot be considered to be the first laboratories, but are in actuality, the offshoots of the clinical laboratories. In all probability these were used by the interns for such tests as blood counts and urinalysis, while the more sophisticated tests were done in the larger hospital laboratory.

The well-documented history of Johns Hopkins Hospital states that during the first year of operation of the hospital, opened in 1889, Dr. William Osler, physician in chief, established a clinical laboratory. In this laboratory "routine examinations were carried out, especial attention being given to the search for malarial parasites in the blood."[8]

In 1894 the Board of Trustees of the hospital approved a recommendation to "regard" the pathological department as a department of the hospital, and to approve a resident pathologist. Dr. Simon Flexner received this appointment.

Dr. Osler, in answer to an inquiry from a Miss Mary Eaton, said he considered a new clinical laboratory the greatest need of the hospital. A gift of $10,000 from the estate of her sister, Susan M. Eaton, made the construction possible, and the laboratory opened in 1896. Dr. Henry Hurd, superintendent of the hospital, wrote in his report: "No more convenient or serviceable clinical laboratory has been erected in connection with any hospital or medical school."[8] A comment concerning this statement appears in the history of Johns Hopkins Hospital. "This generalization of Dr. Hurd may seem somewhat sweeping now but it was no doubt true at the time it was made, for one must remember that in the United States at least, the microscope had been slow in making its way into the clinic."[8]

A statement by Hirsch,[6] describing the condition of laboratory medicine in Chicago in 1890, adds credence and strength to that of Dr. Hurd: "There were no paid pathologists and only crude beginnings of the use of laboratory methods in clinical diagnosis."

Apparently some objections to hospital clinical laboratories were being expressed. An attempt to dispel these objections was made by Camac.[10] He classified the objections into four major groups:

9

1. Laboratories are scientific luxuries.
2. They require space.
3. They are expensive.
4. Clinical tests are too time-consuming.

Minor objections were the fear that patients might drink some of the poisonous laboratory reagents and that some of the staff members might appropriate laboratory apparatus. Camac answered one objection by saying that the hospital lab is not expensive because "the maintenance of the laboratory will be accomplished on $50 a year."

A fifth objection to these ward laboratories was that they required too much time. The complaints of the interns bear a marked resemblance to those of our students today. "New subjects . . . were added to his requirements, but the length of the curriculum, was not increased commensurately with this increase; consequently his medical course was a feast of reason, a large proportion of which he was gulping down and never digesting. . . . the work of today in hospitals is far greater than that of ten years ago, but the intern staff has not been increased commensurately with the increase of work." Camac suggests that in the large hospital there should be a bacteriologist intern, and a clinical microscopist, and a chemical intern. "This position in small hospitals could be combined in one intern." This may well have been the first instance in which hospital interns were expected to do the laboratory "work-up" on their patients. Certainly this remained a part of the intern's responsibility for many years, and indeed, may still be a requirement in some hospitals today.

By 1908 *A Manual of Clinical Diagnosis* had been published. The author, James C. Todd, considered a "kitchen table with a few shelves for bottles, screened off in a corner of the office" sufficient for a laboratory.[11] The sixth edition of the book was the joint effort of Dr. Todd and Dr. Arthur Sanford and was published in 1927 under the title, *Clinical Diagnosis by Laboratory Methods*. This book became the standard reference for laboratories and remained as such for many years. After the deaths of the authors other pathologists edited the text. It presently appears under the editorship of Davidsohn and Henry.

One of the first official references to laboratory workers is found in the 1900 census which listed 100 technicians, all male, employed in the United States. These were not all medical technicians, but included some dental and industrial workers. The numbers of technicians had increased to 3,500 by 1920, with 2,000 of these female. It is interesting to note that in 1922, 3,035 hospitals reported they had clinical laboratories.[12] Despite the increase in numbers of technicians, doctors were still doing most of their own laboratory work, and these "specialists" in clinical work were actually called technicians. In the July 10, 1920, issue of the *Journal of the American Medical Association* are two advertisements under the classification of "laboratory technicians wanted." One sought a physician to take charge of a laboratory, a man capable of doing all kinds of laboratory work. The other had been inserted by a hospital that needed a physician qualified in tissue diagnosis.[13]

About 1915 the state legislature of Pennsylvania enacted a law requiring all hospitals and institutions to have an adequate laboratory and to employ a full-time laboratory technician. This law worked a hardship on many hospitals, since there were so few technicians available.[14]

PROGRESS AFTER WORLD WAR I

World War I was an important factor in the growth of the clinical laboratory and produced a great demand for technicians. ". . . Since the entry of the United States into the Great War, calling many of our pathologists and bacteriologists into the medical department of the Army and Navy, the demand for laboratory technicians has still further increased; if the war continues this demand for technicians will continue to increase not only for the laboratories of institutions, municipalities and private physicians, but probably also for the laboratories of the various hospitals in the Army and Navy and possibly even for the cantonments in this country and the hospitals abroad."[14]

Some practicing physicians with knowledge of laboratory work began to teach their assistants to do some of the tests for them. These assistants often were the persons most readily available for recruitment—nurses and secretaries. Hospitals began to demand physicians with interest in laboratory techniques to run their laboratories, and physicians realized the desirability of relinquishing their work to these laboratories. These demands for laboratory service and more readily available tests greatly influenced the first formal organization of medical technology education. It is not surprising to find that the training programs to prepare people to work in clinical laboratories were established in hospitals under the direction of pathologists.

So far as can be determined one of the first schools for training laboratory workers was established at the University of Minnesota.[15] A course bulletin titled "Courses in Medical Technology for Clinical and Laboratory Technicians" was issued in 1922. Certainly this university was the first to offer a degree level program. This program had the same admission requirements as those for an arts and sciences degree. The exact date this program was set up is lost, but it is believed to be 1923. It is known that from 1922 to 1926 there were 13 graduates. Students there in 1927 learned to do 10 different chemical determinations.* The school has been in continuous existence and is presently approved for 60 students.

In 1921 the Denver Society of Clinical Pathologists was organized. When pathologists outside Denver joined, it became the Colorado society. Texas and Ohio also had state societies. The Colorado society sent out a questionnaire to all persons in the directory of the American Medical Association who indicated they limited their practice to clinical pathology. They were asked for reactions to the establishment of a national society, the organizational meeting to be held in St. Louis at the time of the 1922 American Medical Association meeting. Dr. George Ives, the first pathologist to respond to the questionnaire, was asked to act as a committee of local arrangements. He called the meeting to order with these words: "I have assumed the honor of calling to order what is destined to become the first successful meeting of clinical pathologists."[16] By 1936 they had established the American Board of Pathology and had defined the requirements of the specialty.

INFLUENCE OF WORLD WAR II

Once again a war had a marked effect on laboratory medicine. The use of blood increased, and the "closed system" of blood collection was widely adopted. Although the methods for determining the Rh factor were still crude, this test was added to the transfusion process. The rapid advance in instrumentation probably produced the most obvious effect. With instruments capable of accurately measuring the intensity of color production, dozens of new chemical tests became possible. The first automated equipment appeared. Quality control programs became commonplace. Laboratory medicine moved into the era of sophistication.

Certainly we have not found a definitive answer to the question, "Where and when did medical technology begin?" But, perhaps this exercise in the search for historical background leaves us with an

---

* This figure is probably of little significance to the student who is unacquainted with the clinical laboratory. It would be difficult to estimate the number of chemical procedures available today. Most well-equipped laboratories certainly do 60 or more *routine* determinations, with others available as special or research procedures. Many procedures that were routine a few years ago have been replaced by more precise methods, or have been dropped because they are no longer considered necessary. (One excellent example of the latter would be the procedure for determining the blood level of a sulfa drug. When the sulfa drugs were first introduced, information on clinical use was scanty. Physicians prescribed the amount of the drug to be given the patient according to the result of the laboratory test. Familiarity with the use of the drug has eliminated the necessity for the test.)

almost indisputable fact: a significant number of technicians cannot be assumed prior to World War I. Nor can we pinpoint the beginning of the hospital clinical laboratory; however, a certain logical progression of its growth seems quite obvious. The first portion to develop was pathology, which was followed in order by clinical microscopy (urinalysis) with a later addition of some studies of blood cells, physiological chemistry, and bacteriology. The growth has continued with increases in size and complexity, and the modern hospital laboratory reflects the efforts and contributions of countless people. Perhaps a considerable amount of credit goes to Welch whose "influence helped to make the pathological laboratory the center of the modern hospital and the medical school." [17]

REFERENCES

1. Herrick, Vivian: The heritage of the clinical laboratory. Am. J. Med. Technol. *3*:53-59, 1937.

2. Fagelson, Anna: *Opportunities in Medical Technology.* New York, Vocational Guidance Manuals, Inc., 1961 (Out of print).

3. Gauss, Harry: The evolution of clinical pathology. J. Lab. Clin. Med. *8*:703-715, 1923.

4. Kracke, Roy R.: The future of pathology. Amer. J. Clin. Path. *7*:347-359, 1937.

5. Vaughan, Victor C.: *A Doctor's Memories.* Indianapolis, Bobbs Merrill, 1926.

6. Hirsch, Edwin F.: *Frank Billings.* Chicago, Univ. of Chicago Press, 1966.

7. Flexner, Simon and James: *William Henry Welch.* New York, The Viking Press, 1941.

8. Chesney, Alan M.: *The Johns Hopkins Hospital and the Johns Hopkins University School of Medicine,* Vols. I, II and III. Baltimore, Johns Hopkins Press, 1958.

9. Jackson, Lura Street: *The Medical Technologist.* Cambridge, Mass., Bellman Publishing Co., 1958.

10. Camac, C. N. B.: Hospital and ward laboratories. J.A.M.A. *35*:219-227, 1900.

11. Todd, James C.: *A Manual of Clinical Diagnosis.* Philadelphia, W. B. Saunders Co., 1908.

12. J.A.M.A. *92*:1052, 1929.

13. J.A.M.A. *83*. The bound volume does not contain the advertisement section. A photo of the advertisement may be found in Davidsohn, Israel, and John B. Henry: Todd-Sanford *Clinical Diagnosis by Laboratory Methods.* 14th ed. Philadelphia, W. B. Saunders Co., 1969.

14. Kolmer, John: The demand and training of laboratory technicians. J. Lab. Clin. Med. *3*:493-496, 1918.

15. Hovde, Ruth E.: A medical technology training program study. Am. J. Med. Techol. *23*:184-196, 1957.

16. History of the American Society of Clinical Pathologists. J. Lab. Clin. Med. *10*:679-693, 1924-25.

17. Fishbein, Morris: *A History of the American Medical Association.* 1847-1947. Philadelphia, W. B. Saunders Co., 1947.

3

Development of Standards for Training

Shortly after its organization, the American Society of Clinical Pathologists (ASCP) found itself involved in an attempt to solve two problems concerning those persons who would be working for them in the clinical laboratories. The first was the obvious necessity for defining training requirements for these people. There was also a need for some means of identifying those persons who had completed training. A plan of national registration (later to be termed certification) was adopted. Ten years after the establishment of this registration, the first state licensure law was enacted. The development of standards for the education and training of medical technologists is found in the history of the Board of Registry.

The first report we find in the literature referring to the training of technicians was made by Dr. John Kolmer, a Philadelphia pathologist, in 1918.[1] He had begun a program of training technicians because of the Pennsylvania law requiring every hospital laboratory to have a full-time technician. At the time of his report the program had been in operation for two years and had trained 75 young women. The instruction in preparation of media, preparation of tissues for the pathologist, sterilization of glassware, etc., was given "5 or 6 days in the week and for 4 to 6 hours per day." After completion of this course of study and successful passing of an examination, the students then took "clinical pathology." This included chemical and

14

microscopic examination of urine, blood, gastric contents, and feces and clinical bacteriology. The time required to complete the training is not stated. After experience in a laboratory other than Dr. Kolmer's the student could return for advanced pathology. This included instruction in the Wassermann reaction (a complicated test for syphilis which Kolmer had modified), water and milk bacteriology, "preliminary tests" for blood transfusions, and chemical methods for determination of blood sugar and blood urea. He concluded his article with this paragraph:

> In order to meet the increasing demands for laboratory technicians it is hoped that laboratories with ample facilities and material, will offer adequate and comprehensive courses of instruction and an abundance of practical work to small classes of properly qualified persons, in order to supply the demand for broadly trained and experienced technicians.

It is entirely possible that this article by Dr. Kolmer prompted the first consideration of the need for the establishment of some prescribed requirements for training. Indeed, he was president of the ASCP during the year in which a report was made on a suggested method to be followed in developing a standardized course for medical technicians. He included in his address this statement: "My special purpose is to ask for an expression of opinion of a bureau for the registration of laboratory technicians; a bureau to which a technician may apply; a bureau to which we may refer. I think this can be developed into a bureau that would be of considerable service." The assembly voted to refer the registration of technicians to the Executive Committee "with power." This committee formed a Committee on Registration of Laboratory Technicians which reported that the need for such a registry did indeed exist.[2]

The first move of the ASCP to improve laboratory service set up the "Essentials of an Approved Laboratory." These essentials were formulated by a joint committee from the American Chemical Society, the American Association of Pathologists and Bacteriologists, and the Council on Medical Education and Hospitals. They were approved by the ASCP and in 1926 were approved by the House of Delegates of the American Medical Association (AMA).[3]

REGISTRY OF MEDICAL TECHNOLOGISTS

The history of the Registry of Medical Technicians is, in effect, the history of medical technology from 1928 to the present. The Registry was established by the American Society of Clinical Pathologists (ASCP) in 1928 for the prime purpose of registering (certifying) those persons meeting certain basic requirements in training and education. It was first administered by a board of six pathologists, these pathologists being listed as officers of the society.[4] Later the board became a standing committee of the ASCP.

The objects of the Registry were listed as:

1. To establish the minimum standards of educational and technical qualifications for various technical workers in the clinical, research, and public health laboratories.
2. To classify them according to these standards.
3. To receive applications for registration and issue a certificate of registration to those who meet the minimum standards of requirements.
4. To register schools which offer an acceptable course in laboratory training.
5. To conduct a placement bureau for registered laboratory technicians.
6. To cultivate a high ethical standard among laboratory technicians in accordance with the code of ethics established by the ASCP.[5]

The second and third objectives, or objects as the ASCP called them, have not changed and remain as the prime purposes of the Registry. The first and fourth were assigned to the Board of Schools. The fifth became unnecessary when positions were readily available, and was dropped. The objective has not been revived, although opportunities for employment continue to fluctuate. The last has undergone several changes and will be discussed in more detail in Chapter 8.

The proposal provided for two classifications of workers: (1) medical technologist, a person with a university degree, and one year of experience in a laboratory and (2) laboratory technician, a person with a minimum of a high school education and six months' experience in a laboratory.*

Apparently some changes were made in the requirements of these classifications. Dr. Kano Ikeda,[5] who was secretary of the first Board of Registry, wrote that the term *medical technologist* was issued "only to those special applicants who met the rigid requirements of the Board and were individually elected at each annual meeting, while

---

* It is possible the proposal for classification of workers applied only to those "grandfathered" into the Registry. We know the requirement of 12 months' training for those receiving training after 1928 was added, but the two classifications remained. Williams was registered in February, 1933, before the first examination. She had a college degree, and 18 months' training in a hospital, but received the classification of laboratory technician.

the former (laboratory technician) was given out to all technicians who met the minimum requirements without the examination.'' The medical technologist was expected to have contributed to the field of laboratory medicine through research, teaching, or scientific endeavors which were not further defined.

The Board had little or no information as to the numbers and kinds of institutions already providing some type of training for medical technicians. In order to identify these institutions, a questionnaire was mailed to ASCP members, to hospitals approved for internship by the AMA, and to nonmember pathologists and others not falling into these categories, a total of 862. Dr. Ikeda[5] reported the results in 1931. He found there were 136 courses being conducted in the 400 institutions that returned the questionnaires. He concluded that the training of technicians was being undertaken by universities and colleges, hospital laboratories, public health laboratories, private laboratories, and commercial schools (proprietary schools conducted primarily for profit), and that the courses of study in the last three were generally not acceptable for certification.

In 1933 the first list of approved schools was published.[6] The pretechnical requirements were increased to one year of college with work in chemistry and biology. The work done to earn the diploma received by the registered nurse could be used as a substitute for this year of college. Applicants for registration were not required to take the year of training in an approved school. The 34 schools on the approved list showed considerable variation in their admission requirements.

The ultimate aim of the Board of Registry[7] was to persuade as many colleges and universities as possible to include a four year course in medical technology leading to a degree, or a two year course leading to a certificate. The suggested curriculum for the de-

TABLE 3-1. Admission Requirements of First Approved Schools

Pretechnical requirements	Number of schools
Degree	5
2 years college	6
1 year college	11
High school	7
R. N. diploma	1
High school or college graduate	1

Two had programs leading to a degree, and the requirements of one could not be interpreted. The training period varied from 12 to 18 months.

gree program included two years of work essentially the same as the premedical program, the third year, study in basic medical sciences, and the fourth, in practical service in a clinical laboratory. The curriculum proposed for the two year program suggested that the first year include work equivalent to the college requirements in biology, chemistry, and bacteriology and that the second year be spent in a clinical laboratory.

The 45 years since the publication of this recommendation saw a gradual move toward the acceptance of these two curricula. See Chapter 5 for a description of the first program. The second program is essentially the same as that for the medical laboratory technician. See Chapter 10.

The first five years the Registry was in existence all applicants who met the educational requirements were registered without examination under the "grandfather" clause. The educational requirements were graduation from high school or a diploma from a school of nursing. For those who received training after 1928 the requirement of a minimum of one year of such training was added. More than one fourth of the first 350 applications for registration were received from nurses.[7]

Applicants for registration were certified in numerical order, with Registry #1 being issued in 1930. Although applications had been accepted since shortly after the establishment of the Registry, no certificates had been issued. According to Dr. Montgomery,[8] second chairman of the Board, the Registry represented such a new field of endeavor that the ASCP had no means to assess the probabilities of acceptance by laboratory workers and pathologists; hence, the first applications were allowed to accumulate until it became obvious that the Registry would succeed. The report of the Board to the 1930 convention of the ASCP stated: "Over four hundred laboratory technicians have been given certificates from our Registry."[9]

After April 1, 1933, all applicants were required to take an examination, and the first was scheduled for October of that year. It was an essay type with eleven questions, of which ten were to be answered. Some of the questions were amazingly simple, but despite the simplicity of the examination, 10 of the 67 applicants failed. This written portion, however, contributed only 25 percent to the applicant's grade. Half of the grade was based on an oral and practical examination conducted by a member of the ASCP in the locality closest to the residence of the applicant. The other 25 percent was designated as "personal and psychological attributes."[10]

It was agreed in 1934 that the pretechnical requirements would be raised to 2 years of college, with emphasis on chemistry, physics, bacteriology, and biology, the effective date to be 1936. For some reason which could not be determined the effective date was postponed until January 1, 1938.

At the meeting of the Board in 1935 it was decided to give the title of medical technologist to all registrants with college degrees, and the following year the Board voted to discontinue the title of laboratory technician. At this 1936 meeting it was decided to require a 1:1 student-medical technologist ratio. The Board also went on record as opposing state licensure of medical technologists. The evaluation of schools was relinquished to the Council on Medical Education, American Medical Association.[11]

A new addition to the Registry designation appeared in 1941. An announcement in the *American Journal of Medical Technology* explains it:

> In order to differentiate the original MTs who hold a certificate of registration from the Registry of Medical Technologists of the American Society of Clinical Pathologists from those who affix the same letters to their names and are thus trying to confuse the public, it is proposed that all medical technologists who are identified with the Registry be urged to write, after their MT, A.S.C.P. in parentheses, thus MT(A.S.C.P.) which clearly indicates that they are recognized by the American Society.[12]

The Registry examination for certification has gone through a number of revisions. The essay type was used until 1946, and for a number of years all examinations were graded by one "examiner" to insure uniformity. The October, 1936, examination had six questions, each pertaining to one area of instruction. The question on blood chemistry was "name the nonprotein nitrogen constituents of the blood." The one on histology asked for the names of two standard staining methods for tissues. The other four were equally elementary.[13] In 1946 a few true-false questions were added to the examination, and in 1948 only true-false and multiple choice items were used. In 1949 the test was made up of 200 multiple choice items only, and this format was used until 1969.

The Registry examination has been severely criticized over the years. Many criticized the low passing grade, which was placed one standard deviation below the mean. The passing grade varied from year to year, but was usually in the range of 105 to 112. An attempt was made to set the grade for each examination so that the smallest number of applicants possible failed by one point. Those falling in the two lower standard deviations (16 percent of the total number of applicants) failed. The items covering hematology, chemistry, and bacteriology totaled 90 of the 200 questions. It was possible, if not likely, that a candidate could fail all items in these important categories representing more than half the training time and still pass the exam.

The format of the examination was completely changed in 1969. The questions were divided into three categories: direct recall (47.5 percent on the November 1969 examination), interpretation of limited data (38.5 percent), and application of knowledge to the solution of a problem (14 percent). The distribution of items in the various areas was also changed. There were 50 questions on chemistry and 40 on hematology, instead of the old distribution of 30 each, reflecting a closer approach to the present emphasis in the clinical laboratory. One category, designated miscellaneous, was completely eliminated. Other changes have been made and more are expected. The number of questions in each category is less rigid. Questions on management, virology, nuclear medicine, etc., have been added. The passing grade will no longer be a cumulative total, but a grade for each subject area will be established. Another change has been a marked decrease in the number of examination centers, these being cut in 1969 from a high of 300 to 140. In 1974 a list of permanent examination centers was published. Only a few states have more than one center, and some states do not have any.

The reasons for the 1969 changes were summarized as follows: "a major purpose of any certification examination is to admit qualified persons to a profession while excluding those persons who are not yet qualified. To the extent that the medical technology examination is strengthened, it performs this dual function in an improved manner."[14] This statement continues to apply.

The next major change will be to analyze all questions on the basis of Bloom's taxonomy.[15] Preliminary efforts to do this had been made when the questions were divided into the three categories of recall, interpretation, and application. Questions will now be categorized into the areas of knowledge, comprehension, application, analysis, and evaluation. Questions that require synthesis will not be included. The level of difficulty will be determined also. The expected outcome of the analysis will be a list of objectives of content. These changes will lead to more uniformity of instruction in the schools of medical technology.

It was announced that a change in scoring would occur in the August 1978 exam.[16] Passing scores would be based on "predetermined absolute standards of acceptable performance." This was to be the first step in changing from norm-referenced testing (the candidate's achievement in comparison with all other candidates) to complete criterion referenced testing (the candidate's performance measured against predetermined standards).

A later announcement indicated that research, with statistical data, had predicted a sufficient number of potential problems with the criterion-referenced testing so that the Board decided to continue with norm-referenced testing for the August 1978 cycle.

The first participation of medical technologists in the conduct of the business of the Registry occurred in 1940 when the Board sponsored an amendment to the bylaws of the ASCP to appoint five medical technologists to attend one meeting each year as observers. Two of these were to be appointed from the American Society of Medical Technologists (ASMT) and three from certificate members at large.[11] The two ASMT members appointed were the president and the president-elect. At the June, 1943, meeting the past president of ASMT participated as a member at large, and was a holdover, since she* had served in a like capacity while president. This set the pattern of ASMT representation. In 1946 the number of ASMT representatives was increased to three. The ASMT empowered the president and the president-elect to choose the third member. The two officers selected the past president, since she had previously been on the Board. The Registry Board passed a resolution in 1947 making the three representatives of ASMT members of the Board with full voting rights. The necessary changes in the ASCP constitution and bylaws were made in 1949.

It is presumed that the members at large were dropped when this change was made. ASMT revised its bylaws so that the president, the past president, and the president-elect continued to represent ASMT on the Board.

A change in the bylaws proposed prior to the 1952 ASMT meeting would have required the members of the Board to have had teaching experience.[17] It was argued that such members would be better prepared to advise on matters pertaining directly to the training schools. The arguments against the proposal were that the members of the Board represented the society and should be familiar with the general problems of medical technologists and that they should not limit their interests to training schools only. This proposed amendment was defeated. In 1959 the ASCP constitution and bylaws were revised to allow a fourth member to serve on the Board. This member, required by ASMT to have had teaching experience, was first elected in 1960 for a five year term.

---

* *She* is used intentionally, since all presidents who served during the early years of ASMT were women.

In 1969 the ASMT replaced the president and president-elect as members of the Board of Registry. The demands placed on these officers by a growing, dynamic organization made it increasingly difficult for them to serve effectively on the Board. An additional member was elected according to the changes in the ASCP bylaws allowing five medical technologists to serve on the Board. In 1970 two representatives were elected, one of these replacing the past president. All representatives must have had teaching experience.

In 1977 the composition of the Board of Registry was changed, and now includes six pathologists, six medical technologists, two lay persons, and a representative from each of six participating organizations of laboratory specialists. These organizations include the American Academy of Microbiology, the American Society of Hematology, the American Society of Cytology, the American Association of Blood Banks, the National Registry of Clinical Chemistry, and the National Society of Histotechnology. The medical technologists are appointed to the Board by ASCP.

From its inception the Board of Registry had required re-registration of all persons holding the certificate. The registration fee entitled the registrant to a subscription to the *Technical Bulletin* and a dated seal for his certificate.

In 1968 the Department of Justice questioned the process of registration. It was ruled that registration indicates a certification of the fulfillment of certain requirements in education and training and as such is permanent. Re-registration was therefore discontinued, a new certificate was designed, and publication of the *Technical Bulletin* ceased, all as of January, 1970. The office was moved from Muncie, Indiana, to the ASCP offices in Chicago. The 1978 Board of Registry has indicated they plan to develop and implement examinations for recertification.[16]

The changes in registration regulations created many problems. One was financial, since the fee charged for re-registration provided funds for assistance in presenting workshops and seminars, for the preparation of recruitment material, and for the support of the National Committee for Careers in the Medical Laboratory (no longer in existence). The Board appealed to technologists to send the usual fee to maintain an up-to-date list of registered technologists. A price list of recruitment brochures appeared. Many technologists appear to be confused over their responsibilities to the Registry. The use of the term *certification* as opposed to *registration* is confusing to many (see below).

It would be expected that as the ASMT continues to gain recognition and strength it will move toward exercising its prerogative to represent medical technology in all areas. One such area will be the maintenance of control over entrance requirements to the profession. The ultimate goal should be an autonomous Registry of Medical Technologists. For, as Ikeda wrote: "He (the medical technologist) should be recognized as the master of his own professional destinies and given freedom to establish his own professional standards and define his qualifications."[18]

REGISTRATION, CERTIFICATION, AND LICENSURE

)Until recently the term *registered* has been used to indicate the completion of prescribed academic and training requirements, plus a satisfactory score on an examination. A much more appropriate term is *certification,* the one now being used.

Perhaps it is not too surprising that the term *registered* was suggested in the original proposal. Requirements relative to training were being established for persons who would, for the most part, be working in a hospital setting. "Registered" nurses were to be found in the same setting. Between 1903 when the first states licensed nurses and 1920, 47 states had enacted licensing laws. This precedent

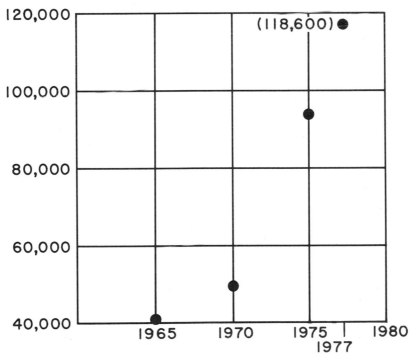

Figure 3-1. *Chart showing the increase in the number of medical technologists certified by the Registry of Medical Technologists (ASCP) from 1965 through 1977.*

23

of registration, with which the pathologists were entirely familiar, undoubtedly influenced the phraseology of the proposal. Perhaps it was anticipated that such registration would preclude the necessity for state licensure laws. The Registry of Medical Technologists, interpreted in a very literal sense, is nothing more than a listing of certified laboratory workers. The increase in the number of medical technologists is illustrated graphically in Figure 3-1. As of February, 1978, there were 120,273 registered medical technologists.

Neither registration nor certification has any relationship to licensure or accreditation. *Accreditation* refers to approval of a program by an appropriate agency. Medical technology programs are presently accredited by the Committee on Allied Health Education and Accreditation of the American Medical Association. Proprietary schools maintain their own accrediting agency.

Licensure is enacted by legislation at the local or state level. The principal objective of the law is the protection of the public through control of entrance into the profession and enforcement of standards of practice. Usually there is an examination of the applicant's credentials to determine whether he meets the requirements for education, experience, and character. If licensure is compulsory, a person who is not properly licensed is prohibited by statute from working in the profession. If the licensure is voluntary, only licensed persons can use a particular title or designation. Others may work in the occupation so long as they do not use the title. An example of this would be the title *licensed practical nurse*. Nonlicensed persons may call themselves practical nurses and work as such, but may not add *licensed* to their title.

Licensing boards or agencies may exercise several powers such as (1) give and grade examinations, (2) issue licenses, (3) suspend or revoke existing licenses, and (4) approve schools. In the case of approval of schools the power invested in the licensing board need not be exercised. Instead, the board may accept schools approved by national accrediting bodies.

At the present time there is no licensing by reciprocity. *Reciprocity* means that one state will recognize the license from another state *if* that state agrees to recognize licenses from the first state.

Federal control of laboratory workers is limited to certain requirements of education and training of personnel in those laboratories that receive federal funds. Federal controls and requirements are of increasing importance in the laboratory as federal dollars provide an increasing proportion of laboratory income.

The 1967 report of the National Advisory Commission on Health Manpower[19] states there is an " 'urgent need' for research to develop model provisions for state licensure laws in such areas as (1) delegation of medical responsibilities, (2) interstate recognition of licenses, and (3) grounds and procedures for disciplinary action."

California was the first state to enact a licensure law. In 1923 the State Board of Health began the inspection and certification of laboratories. Certification of both laboratories and technologists was voluntary until 1937. Presently four classes of personnel are licensed:

1. Clinical Laboratory Bioanalysts—may direct multiservice laboratories.
2. Clinical Laboratory Technologists—perform and supervise laboratory procedures.
3. Clinical Chemist or Clinical Microbiologist—requires master's degree in the desired specialty. May direct a laboratory which provides services only in the specialty.
4. Clinical Laboratory Technologist—limited—(issued in chemistry, microbiology, immunohematology & toxicology)— requires baccalaureate degree in specialty plus one year postgraduate training or experience in the field of the specialty.

Other workers such as technicians, aides, and phlebotomists are not licensed by the State Health Department, but the qualifications and permitted duties are outlined.

Limited licenses are issued in biochemistry, microbiology, and immunohematology to those persons who have a master's degree or a doctorate in the specialty, plus laboratory experience.

California medical technologists believe there is a direct relationship between its strict licensing law and the difficult examinations and the highest salary levels in the United States. Furthermore, they believe that "financial and professional advantages attract high caliber college and university students into the field."[20] Their general comment is: "It works!"

Many other states have laws regulating the practice of medical technology. Students and graduates interested in licensure requirements in a specific state are advised to contact the State Department of Health.

REFERENCES

1. Kolmer, John: The demand and training of laboratory technicians. J. Lab. Clin. Med. *3:*493-496, 1918.
2. Notices. J.A.M.A. *90:*980, 1928.
3. Constitution of the American Society of Clinical Pathologists. Amer. J. Clin. Path. *1:*483-488, 1931.

4. Minutes ASCP. J. Lab. Clin. Med. *14:*491-494, 1929.

5. Ikeda, Kano: Survey of training schools for laboratory technicians. Amer. J. Clin. Path. *1:*467-476, 1931.

6. List of approved schools. Amer. J. Clin. Path. *3:*104-106, 1933.

7. Ikeda, Kano: Twelve years of the Registry and its contribution to medical technology. Amer. J. Med. Technol. *6:*222-234, 1940.

8. Montgomery, Lall G.: Personal communication.

9. Report of Board of Registry. Amer. J. Clin. Path. *1:*111, 1931.

10. News and notices. Amer. J. Clin. Path. *3:*175, 1933.

11. Montgomery, Lall G.: A short history of the Registry of Medical Technologists. Presidential address. ASCP, 1967.

12. News and Announcements. Am. J. Med. Technol. *7:*41, 1941.

13. News and Announcements. Am. J. Med. Technol. *3:*30-31, 1937.

14. Joyce, Harold, and John R. Noak: How the new medical technologist examination was planned and developed. Lab. Med. *1 (5):*26-29, 1970.

15. Bloom, Benjamin S. (ed.): *Taxonomy of Educational Objectives.* New York, David McKay Co., Inc., 1956.

16. Wiler, Merilyn: Board of Registry and certification (Editorial). Lab. Med. *9:*8-10, 1978.

17. Proposed changes in constitution and by-laws. Am. J. Med. Technol. *18:*96-97, 1952.

18. Ikeda, Kano: The present trends in medical technology. Am. J. Med. Technol. *17:*81-87, 1951.

19. National Advisory Commission on Health Manpower: Quoted by Curran, W. J., in Public Health and the law. Amer. J. Pub. Health *58:*1276-1277, 1968.

20. Spence, H. A. and Bering, N. M.: Credentialing in the clinical laboratory sciences. Am. J. Med. Technol. *44:*393-397, 1978.

SUGGESTED READINGS

Roemer, Ruth: Trends in licensure, certification and accreditation: Implications for health-manpower education in the future. J. Allied Health *3:*26-33, 1974.

Stevens, Berenice: State licensing in your laboratory? ASMT News *5:*4, 1969.

Credentialing Health Manpower: U. S. Department of Health, Education and Welfare (DHEW Publication No. (OS) 77-50057, 1977.

4

Accrediting Agencies

The Board of Schools of the American Society of Clinical Pathologists ceased to exist on December 31, 1973. A new independent agency, the National Accrediting Agency for Clinical Laboratory Sciences, was incorporated in October, 1973, and assumed the duties of the Board on January 1, 1974. Because the history of the Board of Schools is such an integral part of the development of ASCP-related and AMA approved educational programs, the chapter on the Board of Schools in the first edition is included here without changes except for the removal of the paragraph outlining the proposed changes, now accomplished, in the structure of the Board.

BOARD OF SCHOOLS

Requirements for the education and training of medical technologists are fairly specific. Yet the means of satisfying the requirements vary a great deal in both the academic institutions and the hospitals, as shown by the several arrangements of academic programs and the lack of uniformity of patterns of hospital instruction.

In Chapter 3 we read that the inspection of hospital schools of medical technology had been relinquished by the Board of Registry to the Council of Medical Education of the American Medical Association. The number of schools had increased to almost 400 by 1949, and the Council concluded it could not continue to do the inspections. It appealed to the ASCP for assistance, and as a result of this appeal the ASCP established the Board of Schools as a standing committee. The first board consisted of six pathologists who were given the assignment to "study the status of training of medical technologists in approved schools."[1]

The first duty assumed by the new board was to make arrangements for the inspection of schools. This was accomplished by asking a pathologist to inspect a school in a nearby town. This inspection was often a cursory effort. The first inspection of the school in which Williams was teaching supervisor took place behind the closed door of the pathologist's office. So far as could be determined, the forms to be completed were filled out over a friendly cup of coffee. The inspector made no effort to look at records or equipment or to question either instructors or students.

In all probability this kind of situation was not unique. A few years after the Board of Schools was organized, a pilot study was conducted in which a medical technologist accompanied the pathologist on the inspection visit. Their reports were filed independently, and in almost every instance the medical technologist was much more critical than the pathologist. Following this study, a medical technologist became a permanent member of the inspection team.

The bylaws of the American Society of Clinical Pathologists were amended in 1952 to allow three representatives of the American Society of Medical Technologists to sit on the board as voting members. In 1960 a fourth medical technologist was added, and the fifth in 1969. A representative was elected at the annual meeting of the ASMT and served a term of five years.

Arranging for the inspections was a most time-consuming task for the secretary to the chairman of the Board. Each school was inspected every five years, the first visit coming within one year after first approval was granted. This meant that approximately 160 schools, or one fifth of the total of nearly 800 schools, must be inspected each year. No money was available for compensation, so that the pathologist not only gave his time but also furnished his own transportation. In well-populated areas this was not an unreasonable burden, but if the distances were great and the pathologists few, inspection became a very real problem. The difficulty was further compounded because of the general policy that pathologists do not "trade" inspections.

Many solutions were proposed, but without available funds they were impractical. A paid inspector was suggested at various times. Recruitment of such an individual, the difficulties in logistics, and the astronomical cost precluded implementation of this suggestion. A proposal adopted by the Board of Schools late in 1968 had great merit. Area workshops for inspectors were established, and improvement in the quality of inspection was the result.

In 1969 voluntary contributions expressly for the improvement of school inspection were solicited from all approved schools. The amount suggested was based on the number of students for which the school was approved, with $100 the maximum requested. In 1974 the amount was raised to $175 for each school. The funds collected were to be used for the workshops and as soon as practical for partial compensation of the inspector's expenses. Better inspection was the intermediate goal, with inspection by a paid professional team the ultimate goal.

The Board of Schools was a body without power: it could recommend, but not enforce its recommendations. The reports of an inspection by the technologist and the pathologist, together with their recommendations, were reviewed by the chairman and such board members as he deemed necessary. The recommendation for approval of a new school, continued approval, or disapproval of an existing school was forwarded to the Council on Medical Education of the American Medical Association. The letter of approval, or notice of disapproval with reasons therefore, was sent from the Council.

Since 1949 the Board of Schools was responsible for establishing the academic course requirements and the essentials for the hospital portion of the program of approved schools. If changes were proposed in the academic requirements, a revision in the essentials had to be submitted for approval. The revision was first submitted to the Board of Directors of the American Society of Clinical Pathologists. If approved by them, it was submitted to the delegates of the ASCP convention and then to the house of delegates of the American Medical Association. It was also sent to the house of delegates of the American Society for Medical Technology. Disapproval by the ASMT did not preclude the possibility of adoption by the ASCP and AMA, or vice versa.

Two major changes in the essentials that were adopted applied to all schools approved after 1968. The minimum number of students in each hospital training program was increased from 2 to 10, and the combination of academic work and the year of training had to lead to a baccalaureate degree.[2]

The latter change in the essentials provided an excellent illustration of the complexity of the chain of approval. After approval of the essentials by the American Medical Association, the Board of Registry incorporated this particular portion into the requirements for certification, and the expected date of implementation was January 1,

1971. The date did not appear in the *New Essentials*. The secretary of the AMA Council on Medical Education had interpreted the requirement by date as a change in the Essentials and ruled that the suggested change must be presented to the Council by the Board of Schools. It required a considerable amount of time to get a change approved by all the bodies; therefore, the ASMT representatives of the Board of Schools submitted a recommendation to the ASMT, which endorsed it, that the effective date for requirement of a degree be December 1, 1972. The ASCP representatives then asked for approval of the date by their society.

The work of the Board of Schools increased greatly, especially in the years since 1965. Not only did it set academic and training requirements, but it received and acted on applications from schools for trial programs that involve changes from the usual format. For example, if a school wished to change the training year from 12 months to 3 months in the clinical laboratory and 9 months in classroom teaching, the request was made to the Board of Schools. In this area the Board of Schools acted autonomously. The Board could set such limitations as deemed necessary and gave final approval after all imposed conditions had been met successfully.

The headquarters for the Board had been the office of the chairman, with secretarial assistance supplied by ASCP. With no income being generated by the Board, it was not feasible to perform other functions which would naturally be considered those of the Board.

In 1968 the office was moved to the ASCP offices in Chicago, and an executive secretary was appointed. The first function assumed by the new office was the evaluation of transcripts begun in July, 1970. Each transcript was evaluated to determine if the student met the academic prerequisites for admission to a school for medical technologists. This function logically belonged in the office of the Board of Schools, not in that of the Registry where it had been previously. The Board was also given the responsibility of the preparation of the essentials of all programs leading to certification. The Board, with the assistance of its parent organizations and the National Committee for Careers in the Medical Laboratory, broadened the manpower base by arranging to have some physically handicapped persons accepted for training. The Board of Schools also encouraged the development of experimental educational programs that indicated innovative ideas for clinical experience.

There was no reason for approval of graduate programs by the Board of Schools, since these are academic programs approved by the appropriate accrediting agency. However, students should be apprised early in their pursuit of a baccalaureate degree that opportunities for graduate work exist. The need for advanced degrees for medical technologists has markedly increased as the scope of laboratory medicine broadens. The opportunities for employment are primarily in the areas of supervision, teaching, and specialization. (End of excerpt from first edition.)

NATIONAL ACCREDITING AGENCY FOR CLINICAL LABORATORY SCIENCES (NAACLS)

The formation of the National Accrediting Agency for Clinical Laboratory Sciences (NAACLS) is a splendid example of the few successful cooperative ventures between ASMT and the ASCP. Each of these societies is entitled to three representatives on the NAACLS board. In addition, there are two supportive level practitioners selected by the appropriate organization. The remaining representatives include one supervisory technologist, one clinical laboratory director, one educator from a four year program and one educator from a less than four year program, neither of whom is a medical technologist or a physician, and two public representatives. The latter two may not derive their primary livelihood from the health industry and may not be directly related to the institutional programs being accredited.

The review committees reporting to the NAACLS Board are: Medical Technology, MLT-AD (Medical Laboratory Technician—Associate Degree), MLT-C (Medical Laboratory Technician—Certificate), and HT (Histologic Technology). The NAACLS executive office arranges for the inspection of schools, reports go to the Board for action, and a final recommendation is forwarded to the Committee on Allied Health Education and Accreditation (CAHEA) of the AMA.[3] The Agency evaluates transcripts for applicants to training programs and acts in all matters related to the education of laboratory workers in the various categories above.

Preparation of certifying examinations, determination of eligibility of applicants for the examination, grading of examinations, and issuance of certificates will continue to be the responsibility of the Board of Registry.

REFERENCES

1. Montgomery, Lall G.: Report of Registry of Medical Technologists. Am. J. Med. Technol. *16*:198-206, 1950.
2. *New Essentials of Approved Schools of Medical Technology.* Chicago, American Society of Clinical Pathologists, 1969.
3. Elkins, C. M. and French, R.: A bird's eye view of NAACLS. Lab. Med. *9*:37-42, 1978.

5

Education and
Clinical Experience

The student contemplating entering the profession of medical technology should possess certain qualities and aptitudes. Eric W. Martin[1] has suggested the following qualifications as desirable for any professional person working in the health care field.*

1. Vision. With creative talents, he visualizes important attainable goals for himself, and those he serves. This gives him a basis for planning a productive future.

2. Perspective. With breadth and depth of understanding, he relates himself to his environment and realizes fully how he fits into the total scheme of life. This gives him points of reference and a sense of direction.

3. Motivation. With inspirational ability, he actuates himself and others to take the necessary logical steps toward the achievement of the established goals. This gives him the initiative needed to undertake the tasks that lie ahead.

4. Dedication. With thoughtful planning, he wholeheartedly devotes himself to his professional duties and responsibilities. This gives him the persistence needed to complete each task he tackles.

5. Stability. With calm and patient effort, he persistently, conscientiously, at times, courageously, applies his talents as fully as possible. He takes care not to dilute his efforts by succumbing to hatred, cynicism, fear, or other negative

---

* By permission of the author.

emotions, but attempts to promote good human relationships. Emotional stability gives him quiet dignity which commands respect, fosters close rapport, and makes people attentive to what he says and does.

Perhaps these seem somewhat formidable to a prospective student and are more expressive of the qualities he might expect to develop as he progresses toward his professional goal. What personal qualities, then, are immediately relevant?

The prospective student should possess a certain amount of manual and finger dexterity. Ordinarily this dexterity is demonstrated by an active interest in the various kinds of handcrafts. In other words, he likes to work "with his hands." He must be able to accept responsibility, for often, quite literally, he is responsible for the life of a patient. This is easily illustrated by the daily work in the blood bank where the medical technologist prepares blood for transfusion to a patient, and where an error may have serious or fatal consequences. The student must have intellectual integrity, a high degree of persistence, and a capacity for patient, thorough effort.

With the heavy emphasis on the academic requirements in chemistry and biology, it naturally follows that the student must like the sciences. He must like people. A dislike for human beings enjoying reasonably good health almost precludes the ability to tolerate ill individuals. Although it is possible to work in certain kinds of positions in medical technology where one almost never sees a patient, nevertheless the procedures done in a hospital or doctor's office represent patients, not inanimate objects. Treatment or diagnosis may be based on the results of the tests; therefore the technologist must feel that he is contributing in an essential way to patient service and care. This contribution begins as a student as he learns to apply his abilities and capabilities in the clinical laboratory. He puts into action one of the primary qualities needed—the desire to work in a "helping" profession.

ACADEMIC PROGRAMS

The student must arrange his college course work so that he can (1) meet the requirements for graduation of the institution in which he is matriculated and (2) meet the requirements for certification established by the certifying agency of the student's choice. The preprofessional years of college work should give the student a sound background in chemistry, competence in written expression, an increased understanding of the nature of man, and sufficient sensitivity to the world in which he lives that he will be able to meet the problems of a changing environment.

The discussion of academic requirements and the features of medical technology education which follow in this chapter, and in this entire book, are generally oriented to standards established by organizations and agencies cooperating with the American Medical Association. This orientation is used because there are more of these programs in operation than any other, and because the program features described are fairly typical of all present-day medical technology education. There is no intent to diminish or to ignore the quality and the importance of other schools, accrediting bodies, and certifying agencies. The AMA-oriented system is used because the authors, having been nurtured and employed in this system, developed this information for the use of their students.

The academic programs of universities vary so widely that no typical course outline can be presented. Hopefully every program provides the elements of a liberal education. Certification requires completion of a minimum of 90 semester hours of academic credit prior to hospital training. Courses must include 16 hours of chemistry, 16 hours of biology with one course in microbiology, and one course in mathematics.

Medical technology programs can be roughly divided into three types:

3 plus 1
2 plus 2
4 plus 1

in which the first numeral indicates the years of academic preparation and the second, the period of clinical practicum.

The 3 Plus 1 Program

In the *3 plus 1* program the student takes his year of clinical practicum in a hospital affiliated with the university or college, but not necessarily in the same geographic area. His practicum is under the supervision of the education coordinator of the laboratory, and must be a cooperative effort with the university. The Board of Schools included a statement to this effect in its *Essentials:* "There should be liaison between the college and School of Medical Technology so that the preclinical work is satisfactory to the school, and the practical clinical work, including didactic instruction, meets the collegiate requirements for a degree."[2] The 1977 Medical Technologist *Essentials* published by NAACLS state that "there must be documented evidence of an affiliation agreement, including evidence of cooperative curriculum development and supervision between academic and clinical facilities."

Students in this kind of program often object to the decreased involvement on the campus. Participation in campus activities becomes difficult, or entirely impossible, if distance is a factor. Ordinarily there are no classes on campus, so the student may feel completely divorced from the university.

The 2 Plus 2 Program

The *2 plus 2* program is completely integrated into the university. Recently the term *integrated program* has been used for this arrangement. The students are introduced to the work of the clinical laboratory in the junior year.

In the *2 plus 2* program the university has an academic department of medical technology. The faculty of this department supervises the clinical experiences in the hospital connected with the university, or in one or more hospitals in the community. If the academic staff is limited, much of the actual teaching in the laboratory is necessarily done by hospital staff technologists. The performance of the student is evaluated by these instructors, and these evaluations are transmitted to the academic office for inclusion in the grades furnished to the registrar's office.

In many programs the time in the associated hospital laboratory is decreased and the student spends an equivalent amount of time in a simulated laboratory within the laboratory or academic department. In this type of learning experience there is no wait for less frequently performed procedures since most procedures can be simulated; the student is not pushed aside because of service responsibilities; examinations are likely to be more relevant and more appropriately structured; the level of instruction is controlled; classes can be larger; and if self instructional materials are available the student can proceed at his own pace. He then enters the clinical laboratory to practice procedures under the pressures of physician and patient demands, learns to respect the important role of the patient, and has the opportunity to perform those procedures the student laboratory cannot provide.

Other advantages are that the student retains a certain amount of identification with the university. He can participate in extracurricular activities on campus, continue his social life, and avail himself of the opportunities for campus leadership.

The disadvantages are almost all linked with monetary problems. Sometimes the university is reluctant to assume the responsibility and the costs of providing the fourth year of instruction. There is a duplication of equipment and supplies in the hospital laboratory and the student laboratory. Instructional staff must be provided.

35

There are some critics who feel that the hospital based instruction is deficient. One frequently heard argument is that medical technology required 2000 hours for competency 40 years ago, the numbers and complexity of procedures have increased; therefore, more time, not less, should be spent in the laboratory. So far as can be determined there are no scientific data on which the requirement of 2000 hours can be defended. Rausch[3] did a study of the original 3 plus 1 and the newer 2 plus 2 programs at the University of Minnesota. On the bases of employer ratings and the scores on a national certification examination there was no difference in capability in the two types of graduates. A follow-up study[4] confirmed that graduates from the 2 plus 2 program were "as capable of performance and professional growth" as graduates from the 3 plus 1 program.

The 4 Plus 1 Programs

In the *4 plus 1* programs the baccalaureate degree is obtained prior to training. The degree may be in any area so long as the student meets the pretechnical requirements of chemistry, biology, and mathematics. Some of the universities offer undergraduate courses in professional subjects such as hematology, parasitology, and histology. Others may list their medical technology curriculum in the college catalog, yet offer nothing directly related to the profession, and indeed, may not offer even library materials such as professional journals. In any 4 plus 1 program the graduate is usually responsible for the selection of the school in which he receives clinical experience and his grades from the latter do not become part of his college record. Occasionally, a college or university will have an agreement with a nearby hospital that this hospital will be recommended.

Experimental Programs

There are some exceptions to these general patterns of instruction. The Board of Schools of Medical Technology encouraged experimental programs, and several were approved on a trial basis. NAACLS continues to support this policy.

The present trend in these new programs is toward a decrease in the time spent in the laboratory learning *how* to do tests. Such tutorial teaching is expensive. A continuation of the type of instruction found in the campus science courses is more economical in time, effort, and supplies and should be pedagogically sound. The greater emphasis is placed on the theoretical bases of laboratory principles and on the assumption that once a student is well grounded in principles he will have no difficulty applying these principles to the actual performance of procedures. Such teaching would have the effect of decreasing the exposure to the hospital clinical laboratory, but would not eliminate it. In one school approved on a trial basis, the time spent in the clinical laboratory is presently three months. The remainder of the year is spent on the campus in didactic and laboratory experiences.

At least one university has a study-work program. When the student finishes one quarter of instruction, he works in the clinical laboratory for one quarter; he then returns to the university for further study, and so on.

Certainly, other variants of the basic patterns will evolve as medical technology changes. One suggestion has been made that the student be introduced to laboratory procedures as early as the second half of the freshman year.[5] It remains to be demonstrated whether this plan is feasible and practical.

CLINICAL PRACTICUM

The year of clinical practicum should develop excellence in performance, a maximum degree of self-actualization, leadership and professionalism.

With the large number of approved schools, each operating in a different physical setting, the number of different laboratory practicum schedules for the training period roughly approximates the number of schools. There are no general requirements for time to be spent in each department, but the plan of instruction for each school is subject to approval by the National Accrediting Agency for Clinical Laboratory Sciences. Ordinarily, instruction and experience are provided in chemistry (which may include toxicology), microbiology, hematology, microscopy, and blood banking. In some programs the instruction in blood banking is given at a separate facility. Instruction in special or automated chemistry, mycology, parasitology, and serology is included, and may be separate from, or a part of, one of the departments listed. Some laboratories include work in other areas such as electrocardiography, nuclear medicine, cytology, and virology.

Students are in the laboratory a total of about 2,000 hours, or approximately 40 hours per week for 50 weeks. If they are enrolled in a 2 plus 2 program, the time may be somewhat shorter, since the school calendar is usually followed. The 1977 *Essentials for Medical Technology Programs* outlines the general content of the curriculum to be utilized in the educational program:

> The curriculum must include all the major subjects commonly involved in the modern clinical laboratory. Each course must be fully described including the educational objectives, lecture outlines and schedules, laboratory experiences and/or exercises.

Rotation in the laboratories varies with the institution but follows one of two general patterns. In one arrangement of the schedule all students are in a given department at the same time. This would obviously be difficult to arrange if the class is large. It would be physically impossible to place eight students, for example, in a laboratory section in which two technologists work. The plan has a definite advantage in allowing the simultaneous presentation of lecture material pertinent to the department at the time the student is learning the procedures. The second plan staggers the beginning dates so that one or more students may start in each department. Scheduling problems increase with such a pattern because the times spent in each department may not be equal. Students may spend from 12 to 14 weeks in chemistry, and only 1 to 2 weeks in serology.

Each instructional area includes some lecture material on principles of the procedures to be done, practice in these procedures, outside readings, quizzes, and a final examination. Other lectures may cover procedures not routinely done in the training laboratory and such subjects as management and supervision, ethics, medical terminology, and laboratory mathematics. The affiliated university may impose some requirements in the clinical experience because of academic credit hours being granted.

Medical technology is becoming increasingly specialized, but the student should be aware at all times of the patient and of the fact that the laboratory tests represent a contribution to the care of that patient. This awareness is best developed in the clinical setting through the performance of routine work. It is in the clinical laboratory that the student should be demonstrating those qualifications mentioned at the beginning of this chapter—vision, perspective, motivation, dedication, and stability. He should be in the process of becoming a professional.

Departments of the Clinical Laboratory

The clinical laboratory usually is divided into several departments. Students learn to do many of the tests in each department, learn the principles underlying the procedures, and learn the use and maintenance of instruments and equipment. A brief description of the work of each department is included to give the student an idea of what he may expect as he rotates from department to department during the clinical practicum period.

The descriptions presented here are necessarily brief. It is nearly impossible to fully and accurately describe all of the highly sophisticated technical activities that are conducted in the clinical laboratory. Students who are seeking detailed information about any special area of the laboratory are urged to schedule a visit to a nearby health care facility to talk with the laboratory personnel there.

BLOOD BANK. Blood for patient use is obtained from donors who come to the blood bank, from a community blood bank, or from regional blood donor centers. If donors come to the blood bank, they must be questioned on their medical history to determine if there are any reasons why they should not give blood. Their blood pressure, temperature, and pulse are taken, and the hemoglobin content of their blood is determined. After the blood is drawn, it is typed and several tests for various diseases are performed. A patient needing blood is typed and his blood is crossmatched with blood from the bank. All of these procedures require a high degree of professional skill, and absolutely accurate record keeping.

The blood bank also identifies the factors responsible for incompatibilities between patient and donor and between maternal and fetal blood.

Many banks prepare special blood products or components. These include plasma, packed red cells, platelets, leukocyte preparations, antihemophilic globulin, and a number of other blood products. Although the automation of certain procedures is found in some blood banks, the exercise of individual judgment and professional expertise by technologists remain the prime means for protection of the patient.

The blood bank is the department in which the technologist exercises the greatest individual responsibility. The pressures are probably more constant and more intense than in other areas, and certainly there are many dramatic moments. The combination of all these makes the blood bank a most satisfactory work area because of the height of the personal satisfaction which comes from contributing so directly to patient care.

HEMATOLOGY. In the hematology department blood counts are done—red cells, white cells, platelets, hemoglobin determinations, and hematocrits. Often the cells are electronically counted. The different kinds of white cells seen on a stained smear are identified (differential). Bone marrow smears are studied to determine the kinds of cells being produced in the blood-making sites. This department may also perform the coagulation studies used in the diagnosis and treatment of blood clotting problems. Special procedures such as reticulocyte counts, LE (lupus erythematosus) cell concentrations, and electrophoretic identification of abnormal hemoglobins are also done in this department. The technologist and the student often have a considerable amount of contact with the patient. Blood for the tests must be obtained, often by the technologist, from the patient. A study of job satisfaction by one of the authors[6] showed that technologists in the hematology department exhibited a greater degree of satisfaction with their work than those in other departments.

CYTOLOGY. Single cells, rather than sections of tissue, are studied in the cytology department. One of the principal uses is for the diagnosis of cancer of the cervix, the familiar "Pap" smear. Cytologic studies also play an important part in the diagnosis of lung cancer. The cytotechnologist does all preliminary screening of smears and marks suspicious cells. These suspicious smears, and random negative smears, are checked by the pathologist.

CHEMISTRY. The most rapid expansion both in number and in variety of procedures has occurred in the chemistry department. It is the most highly automated laboratory, but many procedures are still done "by hand." The large and sophisticated automated analyzers now used in hospitals have revolutionized the operation of the clinical chemistry laboratory. In many laboratories the work in the chemistry department doubles approximately every five years or less. New procedures are added so rapidly it is perhaps unwise to estimate the numbers of different procedures done. However, a standard reference lists more than one hundred procedures.[7]

MICROBIOLOGY. Blood, body fluids, excretions, swabs from wounds, throats, etc., are cultured in the microbiology section to determine and identify the bacterial agent that may be the cause of the infection. After the causative agent has been identified, the microbiologist may be asked to assist the physician in selecting the antibiotic most likely to be effective in treating the patient. Selection is accomplished by the use of antibiotic sensitivity tests.

Cultures and smears are also made for identification of fungi, molds, and tubercle bacilli. Some laboratories may also identify organisms by means of the fluorescent antibody techniques. The antibody that coats the bacterial cell is treated with fluorescin and examined by means of an appropriate optical system. The fluorescent outline of the organism can then be seen. This technique may offer the possibility of decreasing the time presently needed to identify the organisms by cultural methods. This department may also include *serology*. Tests for typhoid and rheumatic fevers, syphilis, rheumatism, and infectious mononucleosis are included in this area. Because of the nature of the specimens and test materials involved, automation has not moved into the microbiology laboratory as rapidly as in other analytical areas.

PARASITOLOGY. The technologist in the parasitology department searches for and identifies ova or cysts and adult parasites. Blood parasites such as malaria are also identified in this laboratory.

Descriptions of parasites have often included a classification by geographic area, such as continent, in which they are commonly found. More extensive travel and wars have increased the varieties of parasites seen and have brought a concomitant increase in the importance of work done in this laboratory.

NUCLEAR MEDICINE. The use of radioactive materials in the diagnosis and therapy of many disease states has become a major area of medical progress. In many institutions the clinical laboratory performs some diagnostic procedures using radioisotope-labeled pharmaceuticals and reagents. These techniques call for special training and a fairly substantial knowledge of anatomy, physiology, pharmacology, and radiation physics.

A special certification can be obtained by medical technologists in the field of Nuclear Medical Technology. In addition, there is a certification obtained by radiologic technologists who specialize in this same area. A large proportion of nuclear medicine departments are located in radiology departments. However, clinical laboratories do perform an increasing number of *in vitro* radioisotope studies as the state of the art of nuclear instrumentation and isotope labeling continues to improve.

MICROSCOPY. The department in which urinalyses are done is frequently dignified by the term microscopy. Many technologists and technicians dislike the work in this department, probably because a normal urine specimen is not very exciting. Yet, in all probability, no single test is capable of yielding as much information as a urinalysis. Besides its value in diagnosing and managing kidney disease, the urine examination may aid in the diagnosis of liver dysfunction, errors in metabolism, diabetes, transfusion reactions, and drug intoxication. A urinalysis, complete with a careful microscopic examination of the sediment, should be a part of every medical examination.

Some departments of microscopy include procedures which do not seem to belong in any specific department. Often such procedures as cell counts on cerebrospinal fluid and other fluids, gastric analyses, and fecal examinations for fat are done in this department.

Stipends

Approximately half of the approved schools offer stipends. These vary considerably in amount, with California the only state known to have established a minimum stipend for trainees. These stipends are not considered payment for work performed and are therefore not usually taxable. However, there may be exceptions due to variations in the office procedures of the hospital.

Certification

On completion of his training the graduate is eligible to apply for certification. The Registry of Medical Technologists of the American Society of Clinical Pathologists requires the dates of the training period to be confirmed by the school and the date of graduation to be confirmed by the university or college. Limitations on re-examination are the same for all categories. If the applicant fails in three attempts, he must arrange a program of remedial education. The Board of Registry reviews the program, and if it approves, the applicant is eligible to take the examination again. If he fails again, another period of retraining is required. After three periods of retraining and three examination failures the applicant may not attempt the examination again. Current employment in a clinical laboratory is not considered retraining. Successful passing of the Registry examination for certification as a technologist permits the graduate to sign his name with the addition MT(ASCP).

EVALUATING MEDICAL TECHNOLOGY PROGRAMS

Some information from *Essentials for Medical Technology Programs (1977)* is of particular interest in helping students to evaluate courses of study offered by various colleges, universities, and hospitals.

The laboratory used for clinical experience should have adequate space, facilities, and modern equipment. The student should have access to a library containing up-to-date reference texts and material and scientific periodicals pertaining to laboratory medicine.

The school should keep records of each student's grades and the types of tests he learns to perform. The school should have on file an outline of the complete curriculum for the year of practicum. This curriculum should show the rotation of assignments through the various departments of the laboratory and the outline of the instruction given in each of these departments. There should be prepared specimens, teaching slides, and audio-visual materials to enhance the experiences of the student.

The student should receive a grade for his work in each area of the laboratory. It should be based on (a) technical ability, (b) written examination on the work performed, and (c) examinations on the lecture material.

The hospital school should have at least ten students enrolled. (Some schools which were approved before this requirement became effective are still enrolling fewer than ten students.) There should be a competent teaching staff. The program must have at least one and not more than two program officials responsible for the following functions and duties:

1. Develop, organize, administer, review, revise and direct the educational program. He/she shall insure appropriate instruction in all areas of the educational program.
2. Document participation in courses or continuing education programs which are acceptable to the AMA/CAHEA and NAACLS and have been shown to provide adequate and appropriate training in the area of curriculum design and teaching techniques.
3. Provide a planned program for continuing education including educational methodologies for all instructional faculty.
4. Provide liaison between the educational program and the administration of the laboratory or institution in which part or all of the program is housed.
5. Provide input into all policy and budget matters which affect the educational program and the laboratory or institution in which part or all of the program is housed.
6. Assure the medical relevance of the program.

The qualifications for the program officials shall be:

1. A graduate in medicine who is certified in clinical pathology by the American Board of Pathology or who has education and experience acceptable to the AMA/CAHEA.

and/or

2. A Medical Technologist who is certified by the Board of Registry (ASCP) or has equivalent qualifications acceptable to AMA/CAHEA, and who has a Master's or Doctoral degree and at least three (3) years of experience in Medical Technology education. Medical Technologists who are certified by the Board of Registry (ASCP) without advanced degrees may qualify if they have five (5) post-baccalaureate years of experience in Medical Technology education acceptable to NAACLS and AMA/CAHEA.

The number of students assigned to any area of laboratory rotation should not exceed two students to each full-time ASCP registered medical technologist.

43

Approved programs should have available laboratory equipment and supplies sufficient to provide adequate technical experience in the various laboratory divisions. Ordinarily hospitals under 250 beds are not approved for Medical Technology programs, as they seldom can provide sufficient clinical materials for good teaching.

Students should not be expected to work in place of paid medical technologists. Students sometimes feel they are "used" because they contribute to the performance of routine laboratory work. Ideally, the hospital having a school of medical technology employs a proportionately larger staff because of the additional time required for teaching.

Information on essentials for schools may be obtained from the National Accrediting Agency for Clinical Laboratory Sciences, 222 South Riverside Plaza, Suite 1512, Chicago, Illinois 60606.

OPPORTUNITIES FOR THE PHYSICALLY HANDICAPPED

Students with physical handicaps may become educated as medical technologists, or in one of the specialties. Federal laws assure all applicants equal consideration for acceptance into educational programs. The success of the handicapped student will depend upon (1) the severity and nature of the handicap, (2) the acceptance by the student of his handicap, and (3) the ability of program officials to improvise and to adapt the educational settings and experiences to meet the needs of the student.

The physical handicaps that would require little or no improvisation include hearing loss, cardiac disorders, loss of motor skills compensated by braces, and speech defects. Total deafness or deafness with a lack of understandable speech, paraplegia, abnormally short stature, or a handicap requiring the use of crutches or a wheelchair all call for changes in training patterns.

Partially sighted individuals would find laboratory work difficult. Vision corrected to near normal or normal by glasses or contact lenses presents no problems. The senior author has never had a student with a color deficiency. She did attempt to teach differentiation of blood cells to a medical student with a color deficiency. The experience was highly unsatisfactory to both. The slides being studied were routine stained smears from the clinical laboratory. The student could not explain what he saw, and the instructor could not translate color into any meaningful symbols. Such a problem could have been solved by resorting to black and white photos of the smears—an illustration of adaptation.

The program officials must be willing to provide step stools or sit-down working area, to adjust work loads, or to exempt the handicapped student from certain requirements as circumstances may demand. Lectures and instructions may have to be written out for the deaf student. If the staff of the laboratory is cooperative and the student has a realistic self-concept, most of the difficulties can be overcome. It is possible, for example, to learn to use only one hand for drawing blood from a patient, to reach needed items or equipment from a step stool or with special gadgets, to transport supplies in a cart that can be pushed instead of in a wire basket that must be carried. Frequently the student himself develops a technique for circumventing his handicap.

The handicapped student "who is not overly dependent, who does not make unreasonable demands on the time and attention of other workers, and who does not indulge in self pity"[5] should have no great problem fitting into the routine of the teaching laboratory.

The National Committee for Careers in the Medical Laboratory did a study which indicated that 22 percent of the nearly 2,000 laboratory directors responding employed disabled persons.[8] These persons performed satisfactorily at all levels, and their work records were equal or superior to non-disabled personnel. Nearly three fourths of the workers had received their training after becoming disabled. Pathologists considered ambulatory and cardiopulmonary disabilities less handicapping than difficulties in communication or lack of coordination that made fine manipulations a problem.

In an article directed to rehabilitation counselors it was noted that some supervisors think disabled laboratory workers are often undertrained.[9] Handicapped persons tend to stay longer in a position than nonhandicapped. Further education or experience in the laboratory preparing them for positions of more responsibility is therefore a worthwhile investment.

A bacteriologist who is a paraplegic said, "All severely disabled people need a weapon—and that weapon is a better education than other people have."[9]

Counselors were advised that disabled persons should not be recommended for laboratory training until they have accepted the limitations of their disability realistically. They "shall be fully mobilized for an eight hour day, and should be able to maintain normal working relationships with others, and to accept the supervision and correction of errors inherent in a teaching situation."[9]

The disabled person should not have any unusual difficulties in finding a position after training. He should realize, however, that some employment opportunities may not be available to him. For instance, the severely handicapped person might find the demands of

45

work as the only technologist in a small hospital beyond his capabilities.

The physically handicapped student interested in any one of the areas of laboratory work should visit a laboratory and through observation and discussion with the technologists in various sections attempt to evaluate his capabilities in terms of task requirements. He should also contact the vocational rehabilitation office in his home or college town early in his academic career. Some financial support may be available to him through that office, or the counselor may know of other sources of financial assistance. The potential student who is not easily discouraged and who is persistent but realistic in his efforts to reach his desired goal should find the goal can be attained.

GRADUATE STUDY

Graduate programs in medical technology have existed for a number of years. Most of these provided the student post-baccalaureate work in a special area such as chemistry or microbiology. Many graduates of these programs tended to migrate to industry where salaries were more attractive.

One of the first programs to break with tradition was that at Temple University in Philadelphia.[10] Two programs were started: one designed to train laboratory supervisors and the other to prepare teachers for hospital schools of medical technology.

Early applicants for graduate work sometimes found that the university to which they applied did not consider the work of the hospital year worthy of academic credit and required extra "make-up" courses. This attitude appears to have dissipated somewhat as the number of applicants increases and as graduate schools become more familiar with medical technology programs. Sometimes these schools were completely unaware of the existence of the medical technology programs on their own campuses. The author encountered an interesting example of the reverse of this situation. She applied for a teaching position in a graduate program connected with a medical school. During the interview she was told the medical school had just learned that a graduate program in medical technology was available on the main campus and had been for years, yet they still wanted to establish their own medical school program. Fortunately, communications are now much improved on most campuses.

Qualified medical technologists now have little difficulty in gaining access to graduate education. The prospective graduate student should first examine his goals and aspirations and then attempt to evaluate with candor his academic abilities. At this point he may wish to continue his self evaluation by taking the Graduate Record Examination (GRE).* (As a matter of fact, any undergraduate student who contemplates graduate work, even as a remote possibility, should plan to take the examination while in school, since the scores are acceptable for several years.) A review book available at most college book stores provides valuable practice in both the verbal and mathematical areas. Review in the verbal area should be emphasized, since many technologists score below a desirable level.

The prospective graduate student should also become acquainted with the various kinds of programs available, by writing to graduate schools, requesting catalogs and other information. He should expect to find a multiplicity of degree titles. He should remember that the title itself is of relatively minor importance—the degree and course requirements are much more relevant.

Now begins the task of aligning occupational goals and educational opportunities. Many influencing factors other than academic must be considered: tuition and other fees, accessibility, family problems presented by relocation, however temporary, flexibility of program to meet personal needs, and the availability of financial assistance.

Academic Opportunities

The major areas in which the student will find academic opportunities are management or supervision, teaching, or a laboratory-related specialty. A relatively new field, which should be of interest in the long-range planning of some medical technology students, is biomedical engineering. There is a desperate need for individuals capable of adapting technological knowledge to mechanized laboratory procedures.

MANAGEMENT.   It has been interesting to observe a rising trend in advertised requests for technical directors who have the master of business administration degree. The medical technologist with advanced work in business should have advantage over the person without any technical training. It is not necessary to have a degree in business administration. Graduate courses will make him more aware of the principles of good management, more perceptive of areas of friction among personnel, and more able to cope with financial problems. Other satisfactory programs may be found in graduate studies in medical technology which have an emphasis on courses in personnel relations, management policies, and statistics.

---

* Information can be obtained from the Educational Testing Service, Princeton, New Jersey 08540.

47

TEACHING. Graduate studies directed toward eventual teaching may follow one of several patterns: (1) preponderance of courses in a specialty such as microbiology, possibly with some courses in the principles and practices of teaching, (2) work leading to a degree in guidance and counseling, (3) preparation in technical education to meet requirements for certification as a junior college teacher, (4) courses in administration, curriculum, or higher education, or (5) a combination of one or more of the preceding.

An example of the latter is the interdisciplinary, cross-college program developed at the University of Florida by the colleges of Health Related Professions and Education.[11] Approximately half the courses required for the master's degree are in the College of Education. The other half are selected after conference with the student, and any approved by the Department of Medical Technology will be accepted for credit. These courses are chosen on the basis of student needs and aspirations. The degree, Master of Education, is awarded by the College of Education. This program has the advantage of extreme flexibility and is essentially "tailor-made" for the student. A doctoral program has been developed along the same general pattern of collaboration.

A number of universities offer graduate programs preparing allied health instructional personnel. Some of these have been developed under grants from the W. A. Kellogg Foundation.

At the doctoral level either the PhD or EdD (doctor of education) may be earned. The basic difference between the two doctoral degrees is the language requirement in the former. The differences in dissertation requirements presently seem less evident. The PhD degree generally encompasses basic research, while the "scholarly" treatment of a subject may suffice for the EdD. This statement should not be accepted as universally applicable. Some universities have dropped language requirements in certain graduate areas. Others have tightened the dissertation requirements for the EdD. The college catalog will provide information about the requirements.

ADVANCED WORK IN A SPECIALTY. The decision to take a degree in a specialty involves two related decisions concerning the choices of a major field and a university. The most commonly offered majors are microbiology, biochemistry, or clinical chemistry, immunohematology, and hematology. Some universities prefer that their students work for a doctoral degree, bypassing the master's. The rationale usually tendered is that the time spent on the preparation of a thesis might better be allocated to the research on which the doctoral dissertation will be based. Conversely, a master's degree does provide an intermediate goal for those who cannot budget finances or time to accommodate the higher degree.

The ASMT believes that one difficulty technologists experience in trying to obtain a graduate degree is arranging for time off, since prolonged absence from work for such purposes usually means one's salary is decreased or becomes nonexistent. To solve this difficulty the ASMT and Central Michigan University have collaborated in establishing a "university without walls." Concentrated courses from three to five days in length are offered in many geographic areas and at national conventions, and lead to a master's degree in management or education. This type of program can be found among the offerings of many universities.

Financial Assistance

Traineeships are presently limited in number and availability. Assistantships and fellowships in specialty areas are often available. The academic load that must be carried may be reduced under university policy. The assistance of the financial aid office of the university can be enlisted to secure information of possible sources of available funds.

REFERENCES

1. Martin, Eric W.: The art and joy of medical communication. Address given at the 19th Annual Meeting, American Medical Writers Association, Washington, D. C., October, 1962.
2. *New Essentials of Approved Schools of Medical Technology.* Chicago, American Society of Clinical Pathologists, 1969.
3. Rausch, V. L.: Does 2 + 2 = 3 + 1? A comparison of graduates from two curricula in medical technology. J. Allied Hlth. *3*:5-21, 1974.
4. Rausch, V. L.: Five Years Later: A longitudinal study of medical technology graduates. Am. J. Med. Technol. *43*:1034-1039, 1977.
5. Fruchtl, Gertrude: New curriculum design in medical technology. Am. J. Med. Technol. *34*:601-612, 1968.
6. Williams, M. R.: The relationships among the personality types, job satisfaction, and job specialties of a selected group of medical technologists. Unpublished doctoral dissertation, 1976.
7. Davidsohn, Israel, and John B. Henry: *Clinical Diagnosis by Laboratory Methods.* 15th ed. Philadelphia, W. B. Saunders Co., 1974.
8. National Committee for Careers in Medical Technology. *Breaking down the Barriers.* Undated brochure.
9. Peery, Thomas, and Catherine Milos: Wanted: Handicapped workers for medical laboratory work. J. Rehab. *33*:20-21, 1967.
10. Roe, Ina L.: Development of a master's degree program for teaching supervisors in medical technology. Am. J. Med. Technol. *29*:1-7, 1963.

49

11. Lindberg, David: The need and opportunity for teacher-technologists. Lab. Med. *1 (2):*31-32, 1970.

SUGGESTED READINGS

Cook, Joyce, and Mezvinsky, Barb: Medical technology education, curriculum for the deaf. Cadence *4:*32-34, 1973.

French, Ruth M.: Knowledge explosion and medical technology education. Am. J. Med. Technol. *35:*438-445, 1969.

Lindberg, David, Rodeheaver, Janet, and Williams, M. Ruth: Competency based modular curriculum. Cadence *3:*22-24, 36-41, 1972.

Musser, A. Wendell: Equivalency testing—partial solution to the health manpower problem. Lab. Med. *4:23,* 1973.

Plant, Alfred: Modern medicine and the medical technologist. Amer. J. Clin. Path. *24:*1001-1004, 1954.

Yeazell, Mary I.: Excellence in medical technology education. Am. J. Med. Technol. *35:*428-437, 1969.

6

Interpersonal Relationships

The student entering the clinical portion of his education finds himself in a new role in an environment with new sights, smells, and duties. His status as a student changes as he learns to combine classroom activities with actual work conditions. He finds he must effectively relate to the many people who contribute to his development as a medical technologist.

STUDENT RELATIONSHIPS

The Student and the Pathologist

In some laboratories the pathologist is seldom seen by the student. The pathologist may deliver only a few lectures, turning most of them over to his associates or to the pathology residents. In another laboratory he may be in the working area every day. In either situation he is the director of the laboratory and is entitled to the respect of all students. Since there is not a working relationship, perhaps the best analogy to describe the relationship between the student and the pathologist would be the relationship between the student and the dean of his college. The pathologist is available for any guidance or assistance that the education coordinator cannot provide, but he should never be subjected to the airing of petty personal grievances.

The Student and the Physician

The student technologist will probably have little direct contact with the staff physicians. But, through observation, he should be learning how to cope with the various types of problems that may arise between the physician and the laboratory. He should be learning to act with discretion and tact.

Perhaps the single most valuable skill that the student technologist can acquire during his period of training is that of working smoothly with staff physicians. He should be observing the techniques of suggesting the need for further laboratory investigation of an apparent abnormality, the diplomatic manner of straightening out a misunderstanding, the adroit "handling" of a bellicose personality. All these are facets of interpersonal relationship, at which the technologist must become skilled if he expects to be considered for promotion.

The Student and the Education Coordinator

It is the education coordinator who expects the student to work, study, write papers, do projects, take examinations, and then to start the cycle over. The coordinator goads the student into doing better than he thinks he can and tries to lead him "to the threshold of [his] own mind."[1] All instructors should be accorded the same respect given to the education coordinator. Hopefully and ideally the student is the reason for the coordinator's being. And hopefully and ideally the student responds with a willingness to learn.

The Student and the Technologists

A student is a student during his practicum year. He is not a technologist; he is becoming one. He should regard every technologist as a teacher, being fully aware that some will be better teachers than others. He should have the right to be taught and the responsibility to learn. He has the right to be treated as a human being. He must remember his education is not being completed: it is just beginning. Unless he realizes his working years must be a continuous process of learning, he will find himself helplessly mired in the slough of yesterday's knowledge. Eagerness and enthusiasm are highly desirable virtues, and probably have the most immediate effect and make the most desirable impression on technologists. Most people are human enough to be flattered by questions, especially questions they can answer. Contrariwise, the same people are not interested in answering questions which should have been answered by reasonable attention to reading assignments. In other words, the technologist usually will be happy to answer questions or to indicate sources where answers may be found, but he will not do the student's home work. Interns and residents are a rich source of information.

Enthusiasm to acquire knowledge must be tempered with tact and understanding of the problems of the technologist. The student should be capable of self effacement at times when it seems to be the judicious action to take. The afternoon a request comes to the blood bank for 18 pints of type B, Rh negative blood for a patient with a dissecting aneurysm is not the time to ask for an explanation of anomalous isoagglutinins, especially if the bank has only two pints of B negative blood on hand! The student should "get out from under foot"—retreat to a quiet corner and wait for the crisis to be over. Of course he can use the time to good advantage by getting some reference books and looking up anomalous isoagglutinins.

A student should be reliable, willing, and cooperative. He should realize before he reaches the clinical laboratory that illness is not geared to a 40 hour week. He should expect to be responsible for the completion of any work he starts, but he should not be expected to finish the work of the technologists. He should not expect to receive compensatory time off because he works overtime. He should keep his working area clean. He should treat instruments with care and his supplies with a view to economy.

With even a modicum of attention to these precepts, the student will have no difficulty maintaining good rapport with the technologists.

The Student and Other Hospital Personnel

In his book on *Teaching Tips* for college teachers, McKeachie titled one of the chapters "How to Win Friends and Influence Janitors."[2] Every student should take this as a tip, too. He should try to influence, favorably of course, janitors, maintenance men, nurses, and the personnel in the business office. Every department in the hospital is important, in some way, to the work of the laboratory.

The ASMT *Personnel Relations Handbook* contains a succinct statement on the relationship of the technologist to the members of the allied health fields. It is included because it is equally applicable to students. "Medical technologists should treat all persons in the allied health fields with the respect and courtesy due them by their knowledge, skills, training and position. The field of medicine is strengthened, improved and advanced toward the purpose of optimum patient care through mutual respect and reciprocity of conduct."[3]

A cooperative head nurse or unit manager can make the collection of the blood chemistry specimens much easier. The cleaning people will do a better job if it is explained what can be moved and what cannot. The electronics shop will help get the recalcitrant instrument back in working order. Essential to the accuracy and efficiency of the clinical laboratory is the work of every employee—from that of the hospital director down to that of the man who cleans the halls. Remembering this will make life in the laboratory easier and much more pleasant.

The Student and the Public

Medical technology is about as well known to most people as is Sanskrit. The laboratory is an unknown wilderness where strange tests are done, from which unpleasant odors emanate, and where many kinds of machines are capable of taking in some blood at one end and spitting out an answer of some kind at the other end. Almost the only thing that everyone knows for certain is that whatever laboratory work is ordered is expensive. The student must learn to define his work, to talk about it intelligently. He must begin as a student to "talk up" medical technology, especially to high school students. He must begin as a student to think about career days and science fairs. Students can be much better ambassadors than working technologists, for they have the vocabulary of their peers to "tell it like it is."

The student should be cautioned that to some his status as a member of a medical institution and the donning of a uniform immediately cause some people to endow him with certain new abilities. He will be asked to make diagnoses from lists of symptoms and/or to prescribe for all sorts of ailments. Such temptations should be politely, but firmly, resisted.

The Student and the Patient

The patient arriving at the hospital immediately finds himself in what he is likely to consider a hostile environment. He is given a name tag that he cannot easily remove. He may be put into a room with one or more "roommates" he has never met before and with whom he must share the most intimate details of living. He may be expected to wear the highly impersonal hospital gown which he will find unattractive from every angle and entirely inadequate for the purpose for which it was intended. He may be uncomfortable, ill, or in pain. He is lonely, apprehensive, or even fearful. He is reacting normally to his abnormal world.

The student technologist comes into the picture as one who will do nothing to alleviate a patient's pain, and may even add to it, and who even questions his identity by asking his name. The patient is not likely to extend a warm welcome. The student should be pleasant, but not Mary Sunshine (or the male equivalent). He should approach his work with confidence, and a minimum of bustle, or as one author expressed it, with "conservatism of manner."[4] The student who lacks confidence should remember that confidence and poise are the products of practice. He should not appear *too* casual—an appearance of friendly interest is important to the patient. The patient is entitled to an explanation of what is going to be done but doesn't need a lecture on the possible causes of elevated glucose levels.

It must be remembered that children are people too, and a condescending manner toward a child 7 or 8 years old or older will make the next approach much more difficult. Students should be aware that children are most perceptive, and react—sometimes violently—to any indication of falseness in the technologist's explanation. The child, too, is entitled to know what is going to be done, including the probability that it may be a somewhat painful procedure.

Patients are interesting people to students. They sometimes have fascinating case histories and diagnoses. Often the student is aware of the confirmation of the diagnosis before the attending physician has received it. Two cardinal rules MUST be observed by every student:

1. No interpretation of the results of the laboratory procedures is made to the physician or to the patient.
2. The information learned about patients is privileged, not public information. The student must keep all such information in strictest confidence.

Often one of the best places to hear this confidence being flagrantly disregarded is on the hospital elevators. Apparently the medical jargon is considered sufficient protection. This may have been true at one time, but today the public is familiar enough with medical terms to understand or perhaps grossly misinterpret the conversations overheard.

Recently a friend recounted a story from his own experience. He had gone to a patient's room to get a blood sample. The resident physician was taking her history, and the technologist listened with great interest. The patient had been shot by her husband, and the details of the situation which prompted the shooting were fascinating indeed. Only a technologist and a physician were on the elevator when my friend got on to return to the laboratory. He immediately shared his newly gained information with his fellow technologist. The physician reached over and pushed the emergency stop button, turned to the technologist and pointed his finger at him. Quietly but emphatically he said, "*You* are talking out of turn. You have violated the trust of that patient and of that physician. I am not going to say anything more, but I don't expect to hear you talking about patients again—ever." The technologist admits the verbal chastisement was deserved.

No student should flaunt his knowledge about the patients or his newly acquired technical vocabulary in public. As an example, one teacher tells her students, "Don't talk about parasitology at the dinner table."

Occasionally a patient will attempt to get information from the technologist through subterfuge, indirect questioning, or rarely, coercion. The patient's usual approach is a demand that his rights be recognized. He has paid for the tests; therefore the right of ownership makes disclosure mandatory. Such requests should be automatically referred to the attending physician.

Perhaps a personal experience will best illustrate the use of coercion to attempt to secure information from a medical technologist. The senior author was employed in a county laboratory governed by a board of county and city officials. A city policeman with diabetes came into the laboratory for a blood sugar determination. The next day the mayor, a member of the board, called for the report. The technologist refused to give it to him, even after being threatened with loss of her job. She was fully supported by the pathologist, and the mayor received only the answer, "If she had given it to you, *I* would have fired her."

Most interesting to the student perhaps are the reports of cancer or venereal disease or pregnancy that he may see. Interest is commendable, and curiosity is normal, but the student would do well to remind himself regularly of that portion of the Code of Ethics which states: "I hold inviolate the confidence (trust) placed in me by patient and physician."

Even more important than all of these important patient relations is the principle that should guide every student, every technologist— the patient is the reason, and the only reason, for his professional existence.

PATHOLOGIST-TECHNOLOGIST RELATIONSHIPS

The employer-employee relationships of pathologists and medical technologists in the hospital setting may be unique in the business world. When the clinical laboratory of the hospital is headed by a pathologist, we have an employer whose professional society originally set the requirements for entrance into the profession and supervised the clinical practicum (Board of Schools), certified the graduate (Board of Registry), and now is selecting the persons to be hired and setting their salaries. This degree of control of one profession by another is unusual. To complicate matters further, the technologist may be employed by the hospital but work under the supervision of the pathologist who is not employed by the hospital, but who maintains an office at the hospital for the practice of pathology.

The financial arrangements made by the pathologist are not the legitimate concerns of the technologist, although they may directly or indirectly affect him. However, a basic knowledge of the complexities of these arrangements may perhaps increase the technologist's understanding of these economic problems.

In recent years the most frequent pathologist-hospital contract has been the percentage agreement. The pathologist's income has been most often calculated as a percentage of either gross earnings of the laboratory or adjusted gross earnings, or some variation of these.* Under this arrangement the technologist is often employed by the hospital but works for the pathologist. The multitude of requirements and restrictions applying to payment for laboratory services by Medicare, insurance carriers, and other third party payers, have created a multifaceted and intricate system of billing and paying for the laboratory and pathology services that are provided in the hospital.

Another type of contract is the mutual working agreement. Under this agreement the hospital grants the pathologist hospital privileges for the practice of pathology just as it grants hospital privileges to a surgeon. The hospital furnishes space and nonscientific equipment, but the pathologist furnishes scientific equipment, supplies, and personnel. He bills the patient directly and pays the hospital for the use of space and such services as utilities and telephone service.

A variation of this mutual working agreement is one in which the hospital furnishes supplies, equipment, and personnel. The pathologist bills patients for certain procedures and receives a fee from the hospital for duties related to teaching, for autopsies performed, or for other services not directly related to health care.

The code of ethics of the College of American Pathologists states that a pathologist may not accept a salaried position in a hospital unless said hospital is operated by a local, state, or federal government. The preferred financial arrangement between hospital and pathologist, then, is some type of contract whereby the pathologist receives professional fees for his services directly from the patient.

---

* Illustrations of the wide variations of these percentages may be found in James A. Snyder's article, The chief pathologist: a salary survey, published in Hospital Management 93:47-49, 1962.

Although contracts for pathology services vary according to the type of service expected and the size of the hospital, one of the most common is the lease arrangement. Under this arrangement the pathologist leases space in the hospital for which he pays rent. He assumes all costs of the laboratory operation including personnel salaries, equipment, and supplies. In this arrangement the pathologist is the employer.

A pathologist,[5] addressing a meeting of medical technologists, described the pathologist-technologist relationships as follows:

> At least 3 different types of relationships exist today: the employer-employee relationship where the pathologist is owner of a private laboratory or where the pathologist in private practice operates a clinical laboratory for a hospital; the senior consultant-professional assistant relationship, in situations where programs of research and continuing education in pathology are pursued in university hospitals; and the slightly different type of employer-employee relationship where both the pathologist and the medical technologist are working directly under hospital authority.

> One common denominator applies in all of these situations: wherever medical laboratory diagnostic procedures are performed, the *ultimate responsibility rests with the pathologist*. Pathology is the practice of medicine. Medicine cannot be practiced by laboratories, nor by corporations, nor by non-medically-licensed individuals.

The illustrations of the pathologist-hospital agreements should be sufficient to indicate the complexity of the employee-employer relationships. It is difficult to find a parallel situation in another field.

Much more important to the medical technologist than the details of the pathologist's contract are the working relationships between him and the pathologist. In a recent study technologists listed "good working conditions" as first in goal priorities.[6] This is perhaps another way of saying that the relationships are excellent. There are certain basic elements inherent in these good working conditions.

Every pathologist has the responsibility to provide a laboratory which is physically safe. This means there must be enough room so that work is not done in proximity to potentially dangerous equipment, such as hot ovens or autoclaves. This may be a very real problem in some hospitals where laboratories are poorly planned.

He must also provide sufficient staff and equipment so that quality work can be produced. Economy in personnel inevitably leads to a decrease in quality if quantity is the principal goal. He must, at the same time, use judgment in staffing the laboratory so that his technologists use their background and experiences effectively, assisted by such supportive personnel as needed.

He should encourage his staff to maintain their technical excellence by attendance at workshops, seminars, and meetings of professional societies. Technologists who perform adequately, or who accept more responsibility, should be able to expect monetary rewards, and salaries should be commensurate with increased responsibility. The advancement to this increased responsibility should be based on ability, not longevity. Occasionally a situation arises in which a new staff member is offered a higher salary than those persons already employed. The pathologist should be aware that nothing is more damaging to the morale of the laboratory.

The pathologist should indicate his pride and satisfaction in work well done. He should be prepared to defend and support his staff in any disagreements with the physicians. One pathologist[7] expressed this particular aspect in words to this effect:

> I shall thoroughly investigate every complaint about their work and shall protect them from unwarranted charges from any source, but shall not condone any shortcomings on their part. Any honest error should be admitted to me immediately without fear of undue censure, but no slipshod work will be tolerated, and attempts to 'cover up' mistakes are unforgivable.

The medical technologist is not without responsibilities himself in maintaining a good relationship. The pathologist should expect honesty, loyalty, and diligence. The technologist should always display a professional appearance. He should complete his work with economy of time and supplies, but he should not sacrifice quality of work to complete more numbers of procedures. He should consider himself responsible for the discharge of all duties that fall within his province. He should accept the possibility, and probability, that upon occasion the work day may extend longer than eight hours.

And, last but by no means least, there should be a feeling of mutual respect between the pathologist and the technologist. Until this is achieved, working conditions cannot possibly be "good."

REFERENCES

1. Gibran, Kahlil: *The Prophet.* New York, Alfred A. Knopf, 1923.
2. McKeachie, Wilbert: *Teaching Tips.* 4th ed. Ann Arbor, Mich., Geo. Wahr Publishing Co., 1960.
3. *Personnel Relations Handbook.* Cadence *1:*21, 1970.
4. Duncan, Ralph E.: Technicians and their relations. Am. J. Med. Technol. *3:*81-89, 1937.
5. Russell, William O.: Technologist-pathologist relationships and the role of the ASCP. Techn. Bull. Regist. Med. Techn. *36:*217-220, 1966.
6. Gerstenfeld, A., and F. J. Whitt: The goal priorities of medical technologists. Am. J. Med. Technol. *36:*159-166, 1970. Readers may also be interested in

reading the comments from technologists to be found in the Am. J. Med. Technol. *36:*234-238, 1970.

7. Foraker, Alvin: The supervisor's catechism. Bull. Coll. Amer. Path. *14(8):* 1960.

SUGGESTED READINGS

French, Ruth: *Dynamics of Health Care.* 2nd ed., New York, McGraw-Hill Book Co., 1974. Chapter II outlines psychological and sociological aspects of illness, and the appendix includes an interesting "Bill of Rights" for patients.

Harger, John: As the staff regards the medical technologist. Am. J. Med. Technol. *3:*111-114, 1937.

Heppler, Opal: Relation of the student technologists to the patient. Am. J. Med. Technol. *3:*117-121, 1937.

Hug, P. L.: Medical technology and the human factor. Am. J. Med. Technol. *30:*277-283, 1964.

Improving professional relationships between medical technologists and nurses. Lab. Med. *1:*25-26, 1970.

Wilkes, Ralph A.: OK—Now it's your turn to run the hospital. MLO (Medical Laboratory Observer) *6:*55-58, 1974.

7
Employment Opportunities

Many estimates of laboratory manpower needs have appeared, and some are frankly pessimistic. A careful look at these needs and the positions actually available indicates the possibility of maldistribution of manpower, rather than lack of positions. Florida, for example, has in the past experienced an acute shortage of well-qualified technologists over most of the state, yet some few areas are oversaturated.

This chapter is concerned primarily with the types of employment opportunities and will concentrate on the positions themselves, with only an occasional reference to geography. It must be remembered, though, that the advantages and disadvantages outlined for each type of work are primarily subjective.

The illustrations of laboratory organization are intended as examples only. The patterns of organization may vary considerably because of the physical layout of the laboratory space and the amount of equipment available. For example, if the laboratory has only one spectrophotometer, those tests that require its routine use should be done in an area readily accessible to it. The number of technologists and their competencies may also influence the division of work areas.

HOSPITALS

The greatest numbers of technologists are presently employed in hospitals. The working conditions, the opportunities, the salary, and the experience to be gained vary with the size and type of hospital. The categorizations of these institutions by size are arbitrary and do not reflect any universally accepted classification system.

The Small Hospital

For convenience of discussion the *small hospital* is defined as one with less than 75 beds. A hospital of this size may have a visiting pathologist or may function entirely without one by sending surgical specimens to a pathologist in another hospital. In some instances, a general practitioner or internist may extend his area of interest to include the laboratory and will act as an on-the-spot consultant.

The laboratory staff is small, of course, and would probably have no more than three workers, only one of whom might be registered (see Fig. 7-1). Obviously, all laboratory workers must be able to do all the tests, or almost all. In order for the laboratory to provide emergency services at night and on weekends, the technologists and/or technicians must take "call." This means one of them is "on call" for emergency work after the regular hours of the laboratory. Some sort of compensation is given, either time or money. The latter is usually offered, since compensatory time is difficult to arrange. If the hospital is very small, 25 or 30 beds for example, the person in the laboratory may be expected also to take the x-rays when on call.

ADVANTAGES. Certainly the technologist in this type of laboratory must develop a certain degree of self-reliance. Unfortunately, this self reliance may be misjudged. Since communication is not a problem, every technologist is aware of what is going on. A close working relationship with other technologists can develop excellent rapport, but in case of personality conflicts can become unbearable.

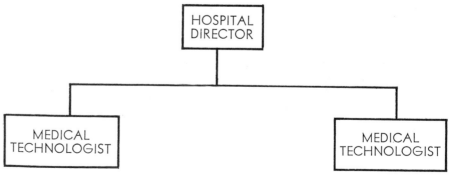

Figure 7-1. *Staffing pattern of small hospital laboratory.*

The salary is often higher than in a larger institution, and with over-time for call duty looks very attractive.

DISADVANTAGES. Many small hospitals are in equally small towns, and the social and cultural opportunities may be limited. Time off for meetings, workshops, and vacations is difficult to arrange. With no pathologist in residence, supervision is nil, and consultation in times of doubt is not readily available. Usually only routine proce-dures are done, and only the minimum of equipment may be available. Although the numbers and kinds of procedures are dictated by the availability of equipment and the qualifications of the personnel, the strongest factor is economic. It is not feasible to develop a proce-dure if it is ordered but once a month.

The Medium-sized Hospital

The *medium-sized hospital* includes those with capacities up to 300 beds. The laboratory usually is somewhat departmentalized, even though the division may not extend to physical separation of the departments. The trend throughout all hospitals is to provide seven-day-round-the-clock coverage, so there may be an evening shift and possibly a night shift. There will be a pathologist as the director, and he may have an assistant. Certainly the hospitals approaching the upper limit of bed capacity in this category should have a chief technologist or laboratory supervisor (see Figs. 7-2 and 7-3).

ADVANTAGES. This size of hospital is an ideal one in which to get a well-rounded exposure to all clinical areas, since it is usually possible to arrange to rotate through the departments. This type of plan will already be in operation in many laboratories. There is an opportunity to advance to department head, sometimes called section chief, with a concomitant increase in salary. There are salary incre-

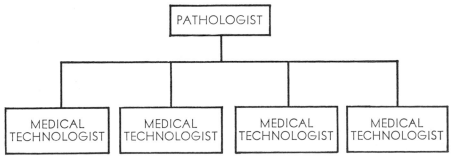

Figure 7-2. *Staffing pattern of medium hospital laboratory with little departmentalization.*

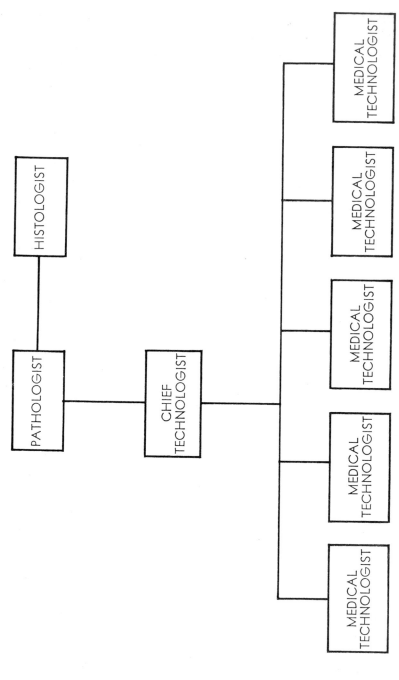

Figure 7-3. *Staffing pattern of medium hospital laboratory with departmentalization.*

ments for those who work the evening and night shifts. If these shifts are omitted, the on-call system will add to the take-home pay.

DISADVANTAGES. Equipment may not be quite as sophisticated, and automation may be less utilized as compared to a larger laboratory, and the number of tests done not quite as extensive or comprehensive. Advancement in responsibility is frequently slow. Rotation of workers on evening and night shifts may be required.

The Large Hospital

The *large hospital* is defined as one with more than 300 beds. The laboratory will be well departmentalized, and each department will have a section chief. There will be a chief technologist and, if there is a school of medical technology, there should also be an education coordinator. There will be two or more pathologists, and in the larger laboratories there will frequently be technologists with advanced degrees in charge of each of the main divisions. Other hospitals may employ specialists to head these departments, such as a bacteriologist in charge of microbiology or a biochemist in charge of chemistry. These are in addition to the section chiefs (Fig. 7-4). The laboratory will have a great deal of automated equipment and may be computerized in many areas. The prospective employee frequently has the opportunity to choose the laboratory in which he wishes to work and thus to specialize. This is the type of laboratory to choose if one wishes to gain experience in depth in one area.

The *chief technologist* may also be called technical director, assistant director, administrative technologist, administrative assistant, or laboratory coordinator. His function is approximately the same under any one of these titles. He relieves the pathologist of some of his onerous duties related to the operation of the laboratory. He arranges work rotation and vacation schedules, orders supplies, sees most of the salesmen, and performs "all the duties and functions necessary to the efficient, economic and quality supervision of the department."* He may also contribute to patient service by actual work in one or more of the departments.

In Figures 7-3 and 7-4, histology is shown as a separate department. Since the preparation of tissue specimens is of utmost importance to the pathologist, the histologist would work directly under his supervision, and the chief technologist may have only minor responsibilities in this department.

The *section chief* is responsible for one department only. His

---

* *Personnel Relations Handbook.* Cadence, *1* (2):22, 1970.

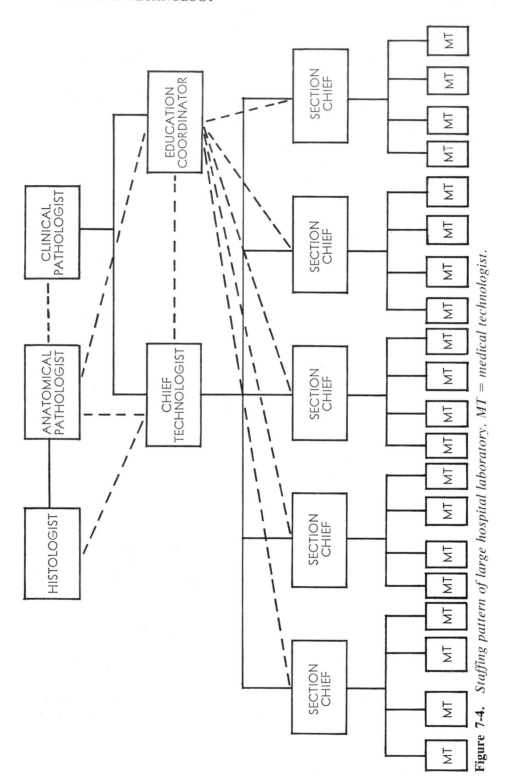

Figure 7-4. *Staffing pattern of large hospital laboratory. MT = medical technologist.*

principal function is to see that the work is done with accuracy, economy, and dispatch. He recommends new procedures or sets up those suggested by the chief technologist or pathologist. If there is a medical technology program he assists the education coordinator as needed and supervises students in their rotation through his section. In the very large, entirely departmentalized laboratory there may be an assistant section chief (Fig. 7-5).

Some larger hospitals have experimented with work schedules other than the usual 8 to 5. One laboratory runs a 10 hour day and a four day week. Another put its chemistry laboratory personnel on a schedule of seven days on, and seven days off. No vacation or holiday time accrues on this plan. There are advantages and disadvantages relating to most innovative work schedules. They can often work well in some institutional settings, and poorly in others.

Other hospitals have started plans whereby the employee is compensated for unused sick time. This time, plus vacation time, is accumulated as "paid personal days" and may be taken as desired.

ADVANTAGES. The fringe benefits available to medical technologists working in large hospitals vary so much it is impossible to state with certainty which will be offered in the above positions. Instead, those listed here are benefits that may be found by the prospective employee.

Since 1951, employees of nonprofit hospitals have been covered by Social Security. More hospitals are beginning to offer some type of retirement plan. This is often in the form of insurance that may be converted to a retirement plan after leaving the employ of the hospital. Hospitalization is almost never offered except under an insurance plan such as Blue Cross-Blue Shield. The premiums of these plans may be paid in part or in full by the hospital. Other benefits that may be offered are laundry of uniforms, lunch or dinner according to the schedule worked, other meals at cost, discounts on drugs, tuition-free university courses, attendance at state and national meetings of professional organizations, increase in vacation time with longevity, scheduled salary increases or merit raises, and free life insurance. Occasionally, a hospital provides rooms or apartments at reasonable rents for its employees.

DISADVANTAGES. Physical separation of the departments in the laboratory of a large hospital often produces a feeling of isolation. The chain of command becomes more complicated, and the problems of communication increase. The opportunities for advancement increase as positions of responsibility are added, but the turnover in these positions may be so limited that advancement may be slow.

67

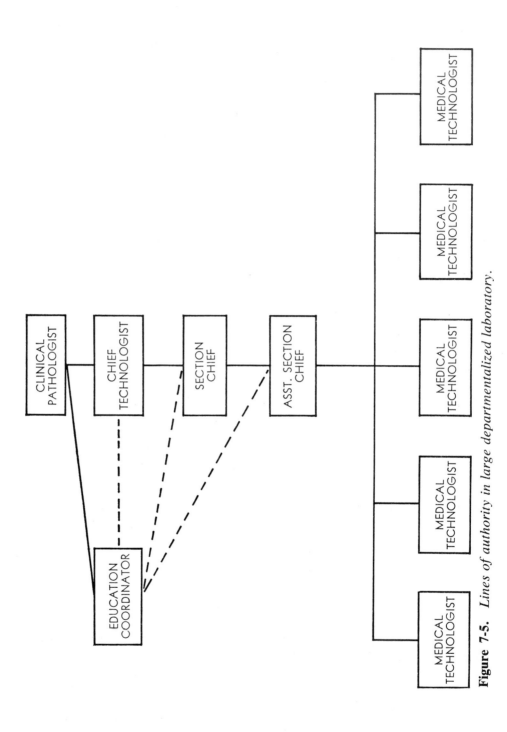

Figure 7-5. *Lines of authority in large departmentalized laboratory.*

Unless there is an overlapping of shifts, there may be problems related to maintenance of supplies and reagents. If different methods and instruments are used on the evening and night shifts there may be problems of quality control. Skills in areas other than one's specialty are likely to become "rusty" or even obsolete.

Opportunities for Part-time Work

The hospital laboratory offers numerous opportunities to women who wish to work only part-time. Often the hours can be arranged entirely to suit the convenience of the technologist. Some women find the night shift desirable, since they can be at home during the hours the children are not in school. If there has been a lengthy absence from laboratory work, the part-time employee may need retraining. Some hospitals are offering such retraining with stipends or even full salary. Retraining may be in the one specialized area in which the technologist is to be working or may be general but usually is in the form of on-the-job training rather than a formal course of study. Few hospitals are willing to commit funds, personnel time, or space to retraining unless there is a serious shortage of personnel, and unless they have some assurance that the retrained employee will remain on the payroll for a reasonable period of time. The length of time for retraining will depend upon the time elapsed since employment, the needs of the laboratory, and the expressed plans of the trainee.

Hospitals for Profit

A new type of hospital has opened in many communities. This hospital is built and managed by a corporation and is expected to show a profit for its stockholders. Many of the expensive departments such as obstetrics, pediatrics, and the emergency room may be lacking. The advantages and disadvantages of employment in such a hospital would be approximately the same as those in another hospital of comparable size. Salaries may be somewhat higher and will always be competitive.

Veterans Administration and other Federal Hospitals

The work in this type of hospital varies but little from that in any other hospital. Since departmentalization is common, experience in the laboratory of a Veterans hospital may be limited to one area.

ADVANTAGES. After a probationary period, positions are secure. Pay raises are automatic, and salaries are competitive with those in other hospitals, since they are "realistically geared to the economy.''[1] Employees are paid under the General Schedule (GS). Technologists without experience usually start at GS7. The beginning pay levels at which the VA and other government agencies hire personnel are often determined by local needs and the law of supply and demand. Federal institutions have a fair degree of local autonomy in adjusting pay levels to meet their own particular needs. In most communities, the VA and other federal agencies pay slightly better than do civilian institutions for equivalent positions. This, combined with an excellent package of personnel benefits, serves to promote stability in the government work force. It is possible to qualify for a higher rating and thus be eligible for positions of more authority. With seniority there is the possibility of applying for positions in other geographic areas. Employees of government hospitals may make purchases in the hospital canteen, and savings are considerable on items on which there is a federal tax. Vacations can be accrued to a generous number of days, and more holidays are observed than at most civilian hospitals. Group life and health insurance paid in part by the government is available. There is a liberal retirement plan.

DISADVANTAGES.　The most common complaint of federal hospital employees seems to be the requirement of accounting for all time spent at work. For example, a trip to the dentist can be deducted from sick leave time, but a trip to see a sick parent must be deducted from annual leave entitlement. Pay is figured in increments of one hour. Some technologists consider the administrative policies in government service excessively rigid and complex. However, once a government employee becomes accustomed to the system, its advantages in the form of employee security and fair treatment become apparent. Government ''red tape'' is tedious, as illustrated by the fact that sometimes it seems easier to purchase a $2,000 item than a $2 one. Many things that can be handled on an informal basis in civilian hospitals require burdensome bureaucratic treatment in a VA or other federally operated hospital.

Supervisory Opportunities for Men and Women

Since its beginning, medical technology has been a profession dominated by women. The single most important factor contributing to the large percentage of women has been the low salaries. The majority of medical technologists work in hospital laboratories, and it is only recently that salaries of hospital personnel below management categories have been raised to respectable levels. Supervisory positions are available to those who have chosen to make careers their primary personal objectives. Salaries for chief technologists are

70

now high enough to be enticing. The young person who is willing to plan his or her future by arranging for maximum exposure to a variety of work experiences and to further his or her educational objectives by graduate work will surely find unlimited opportunities in the hospital or commercial laboratory of tomorrow. The opportunities in teaching are increasing rapidly. These positions are attractive to men and women because of the potential for advancement.

THE PRIVATE LABORATORY

The privately owned laboratory may be a small one in a physician's office or may be run by a physician or a pathologist for other physicians. The duties are approximately the same as would be found in the laboratory of a medium-sized hospital, except that little or no weekend work is done and there is no night or on-call work.

In some states it is legal for a nonmedical person to establish and direct a diagnostic laboratory. Such an enterprise requires considerable financing to begin operation and cooperative physicians to provide a sufficient number of patients. Once established and with an adequate test load, the financial rewards are high, but considerable business acumen is needed to attain these rewards.

Several long-established laboratories in Florida, where it is legal to own such a laboratory, have been bought by large national firms. Similar transactions have been reported in many other states. It is possible this indicates a trend away from individual ownership to a "combine" operation for reasons of mass analyses at decreased costs and increased profits. This type of operation is discussed more fully under "Industry." In some states where it is legal for a non-physician to own and operate a laboratory, it is also legal to advertise laboratory services to the general public, and to perform these services without a physician's order. This type of operation can be extremely lucrative, but is fraught with possibilities of malpractice complaints. Medical technologists who are not prepared to deal with this risk and its attendant legal complications are advised to be cautious in entering into private laboratory partnerships.

ADVANTAGES. In the privately owned laboratory there is the satisfaction of being "the boss." Extra effort on the part of the owner adds to his income.

The technologist who works in the nonindustrial private laboratory can expect a salary similar to that offered by hospitals in the area. There is no night call, and weekend work is usually limited. Occasionally the owner of the laboratory sets up an incentive bonus plan based on a predicted increase in workload and income.

71

DISADVANTAGES. The privately owned laboratory has an unusually high investment in equipment that has a relatively short life span. Adequate, well-trained technologists are vital but expensive. Often such chores as record keeping and ordering supplies extend the working hours of the owner well beyond the usual eight-hour day.

The technologist in a physician's laboratory may be required to serve also as receptionist or bookkeeper. The number of procedures done is limited because it is more economical to refer to specialized laboratories tests ordered infrequently or requiring expensive equipment. There will be difficulties in keeping up with current developments in the field and in arranging attendance at workshops and professional meetings. Vacations may have to be scheduled at the same time the physician will be away from the office.

PUBLIC HEALTH LABORATORIES

Public health laboratories may be under city, county, or state control and almost always offer positions that are regulated by civil service. A competitive examination may be required before appointment. Some laboratories offer diversified services; others are almost entirely confined to examinations in serology and bacteriology. The latter concentration tends to make the work in such a laboratory rather monotonous.

ADVANTAGES. Civil service appointments are secure. Benefits offered all state, city, or county employees are available, such as retirement plans, adequate vacations, and pay equal to or above salaries in competing institutions.

DISADVANTAGES. Advancement may be slow. The hierarchal division of staff according to civil service rating is sometimes reflected in disagreement as to individual responsibility and bureaucratic frustrations such as are discussed in the section on VA hospitals.

SALES

There are numerous opportunities for positions with companies manufacturing laboratory equipment or supplies. Manufacturers now advertise that both males and females will be considered for sales positions, and increasing numbers of women are obtaining these positions. Medical technologists are recruited because a thorough acquaintance with equipment economizes on the time usually devoted to the indoctrination of the new salesman. The expertise obtained in medical technology can be invaluable in introducing a new item into a laboratory. According to Jack Closson,* a medical technologist who spent some years in sales, the qualifications needed besides technical ability include dedication, creativity, diligence, self-motivation, personality, moderated aggressiveness, self-discipline, reliability, maturity, a neat appearance, the ability to organize, loyalty, vitality, concern for others, and integrity.

More than one company producing automated laboratory equipment has hired female technologists to install the instruments and to train those who will be using them. The sales career barriers that traditionally were imposed upon women, for whatever reasons, seem to have been surmounted as the equal employment opportunity laws have been implemented.

ADVANTAGES.   Since most sales forces operate on a commission basis, either full or partial, the optimistic, enthusiastic person who does not mind working hard will find his income is limited only by his ability to sell and his initiative. This type of work is not for the introverted, shy person. There is always a possibility of phenomenal financial success for the optimist who believes in his product. Selling provides a challenge that many other types of work do not.

The fringe benefits in sales are usually competitive with those provided in hospitals. They may include comprehensive life and hospital insurance plans, a retirement plan paid in full or in part by the company, the possibility of paid tuition for academic studies if these can be arranged to fit the schedule of the salesman, options to purchase stock, and the use of a car. Advancement is possible through promotion to regional supervisor or to district manager of sales. From there promotion may lead to sales manager in the main office and on to vice president in charge of sales, or even to president of the company.

DISADVANTAGES.   Frequent travel does not appeal to many people. If the territory is large, the salesman may be home only on the weekend. This requires an understanding, resourceful, and self-reliant family. Children miss the parental influence, and attempts to crowd the family social life into weekends are most difficult. Salesmen are frequently required to represent the company at conventions with displays of new equipment and products. Many of the small conventions are scheduled for weekends, thus further limiting the salesman's free time. The average salesman seems to feel his working life as a salesman is not too long. He is apt to express it this way: "You don't see very many old salesmen around, do you?" If promo-

---

* ASMT News, July, 1973. Quoted with permission.

tion to an area office or to the main office has not come by the time he is 40, it seems a new career direction should be considered.

COMMERCIAL AND INDUSTRIAL LABORATORIES

There seems to be little question but that the movement of technologists and laboratory workloads in the next decade will be from the hospital laboratory into centralized commercial laboratories. During recent years, many so called "reference" laboratories have become established. At first these laboratories performed only examinations that were too unusual or exotic for the average hospital laboratory's resources. The success enjoyed by these commercial ventures demonstrated the feasibility of transporting specimens from hospitals and clinics to large automated central laboratories with economy and efficiency. As a result, many small privately operated commercial laboratories are now being purchased by these larger "reference laboratories" and by large corporate interests already related in some way to the laboratory field. Increasingly larger numbers of laboratory personnel will be employed by these centralized types of operations, and proportionately fewer technologists and technicians will be working in small hospitals and clinics.

The first section of the clinical laboratory of the hospital most likely to be partially transferred to the central laboratory is chemistry. This section encompasses so many of the unusual and sophisticated procedures that only the largest hospital can expect to do all of them. Any tests done in small numbers at irregular intervals are expensive in terms of personnel, equipment, and reagents.

Industry employs technologists for three different categories of work besides sales. Technologists are required for the laboratory that is a part of the health program for employees, for the working laboratory such as described above, and for research. The latter may include the "research and development" department, which is often devoted to such activities as developing commercially marketable forms of packaged laboratory reagents.

Technologists are also employed as educational specialists by laboratory supply and equipment manufacturers. These technologists are responsible for providing workshops and seminars for those who are users, or potential users, of the products marketed by their employers. In some instances the educational offerings provided by these manufacturers are purely educational in content, and contain no commercially oriented material.

Some manufacturing companies are hiring attractive female medical technologists to act as public relations representatives.

Technologists are also employed by these same firms to assist in the teaching of the salesmen. A major laboratory supply house now has a nationwide team of five female technologists who serve as educational representatives for their company.[2]

ADVANTAGES. The pay scale in industry is above that in most hospitals. Industry also offers many fringe benefits such as those described under Sales. There are often recreation parks, social clubs, and other "company" activities. Occasionally there are minor benefits. For example, a pharmaceutical firm may provide free vitamins. Sometimes employees must belong to a union. (Unfamiliarity with unions makes it difficult for the writers to comment on them.*)

DISADVANTAGES. The technologist who entered the field with the desire to be a part of the health team may find it difficult to see the relationship of his work in the industrial laboratory or with the laboratory supplier, to the care of the patient. Of course, those who have little desire for contact with patients may find industry the ideal place to work.

The technologist in industry may find he is "boxed in." Since efficient operation is essential for a profit-making organization, the technologist may be assigned to one type of procedure or to an assembly-line type of work organization where he does only one portion of a procedure, and where he has no direct contact with patients.

RESEARCH

Most positions in research will be found either in industry or in a medical center. Industrial research may be entirely directed toward the search for new products and the necessary testing (bacteriological, animals, etc.) prior to distribution of a product. Medical center research is perhaps more diversified. It may involve development or evaluation of a new laboratory method, a new clinical treatment method, or any of a host of other varying types of investigations. Medical technologists do not usually have the necessary background to do sophisticated basic research without supervision. Hence, the research problem will be outlined by the principal investigator who will delegate tasks and responsibilities to the technologist.

A successful research technologist should have certain characteristics. He must be able to work alone with a minimum of direction

---

* An excellent review of pros and cons of unions will be found in the *Personnel Relations Handbook* published in Cadence, Vol. 1, No. 2 (March, 1970). It is also available from the American Society for Medical Technology, 5555 West Loop South, Bellaire, Texas 77401.

and must be content to have all his work go for naught if the original idea produces negative or inconclusive results. He must be aware that occasionally the timing of an experiment may require night or weekend hours. He must be scrupulously honest, and above all, he must be patient.

Many times students contemplating medical technology as a profession state that their reason for entering the field is to discover a cure for cancer. To be bluntly realistic, a medical technologist probably will not make this discovery alone, but he may make a worthwhile contribution to such a discovery through assisting a researcher with his work. The plaudits may not be many, but the personal satisfaction can be immense.

TEACHING

Medical technology has been much slower than some other health fields in acknowledging the need for teachers who have had educational preparation. Each medical technology program, whether affiliated with a hospital or a university, must have an educational coordinator whose principal responsibility is the direction of student education. The 1977 *Essentials for Medical Technology Programs* require that medical technologists who are program officials must, in addition to being an MT(ASCP), possess minimum qualifications of a master's degree and three years of experience in education. The person possessing a baccalaureate degree may qualify providing he has five years of education experience.

There is a growing trend toward the use of simulated laboratories for teaching. These laboratories give the student the basic principles, theories, and practical applications of clinical laboratory procedures. Such teaching increases the need for qualified faculty. The time spent later in the clinical laboratory provides practice in the procedures, instruction in procedures not learned in the teaching laboratory, and the necessary introduction to the patient-oriented laboratory and its distinctive atmosphere.

Many community colleges are offering courses for medical laboratory technicians and for those who wish to transfer to a four-year medical technology program. These colleges are anxious to recruit personnel capable of providing the necessary teaching. The person with an advanced degree will find a goodly number of openings, provided he is not limited in the geographic area in which he can work.

There are great numbers of colleges and universities that have schools of allied health professions. These schools are in continual need of teachers, assistant and associate deans, and deans. There is no reason why a medical technologist who can meet the academic requirements for appointment and who has the necessary administrative ability cannot fill any one of these positions.

ADVANTAGES, UNIVERSITY.   The reward that comes from the knowledge that you have contributed to the learning of a student and to his ability to represent his profession adequately and responsibly cannot be duplicated. At the university or college level a certain amount of status is attached to an academic appointment. The fringe benefits may include free tuition courses for yourself and your family, retirement plans in addition to social security, annuity plans, sabbatical leaves with pay, and longer vacation periods. Professors are now receiving fairly respectable salaries, and the trend is upward. Promotion in rank and responsibility is possible. A teacher may go through the ranks from instructor to department chairman. From there, the possibility of promotion is limited by the availability of administrative positions and the ambition, capabilities, and credentials of the professor.

ADVANTAGES, HOSPITAL.   The education coordinator in the hospital should receive extra compensation, ideally above the salary of a section chief. A "label" will help too. For example, instead of the name tag carrying the identification "Medical Technologist," it should read "Education Coordinator, Medical Technology Program." Pride in, and recognition of, the position result in a happier, more effective teacher.

DISADVANTAGES, UNIVERSITY.   If the academic load is heavy, it is difficult to keep abreast of all the new developments in the field. A good in-service program and attendance at workshops, seminars, and conventions will help. The academic red tape is sometimes frustrating, and there are the inescapable demands of the grading system. Salaries may depend upon the whims of the state legislature or the state budget commission, and raises are sometimes smaller and less frequent than would be considered desirable. And—students don't always appear to appreciate the efforts exerted to give them meaningful learning experiences.

DISADVANTAGES, HOSPITAL.   Since the instructors are also usually working technologists, interruptions to teaching schedules often occur because of emergencies or unexpectedly heavy laboratory workloads that demand their presence in the clinical laboratory. Classes may have to be suspended until the emergency or interruption is dealt with and instructors are able to return to their collateral duties in the teaching program. Another disadvantage of the hospital training program is that many hospitals have small enrollments in their medical technology course. The small classes, coupled with the informality of teaching and frequent interruptions as mentioned above, make it difficult to maintain a good learning situation.

Student evaluation is quite difficult in the small class situation found in many hospital laboratories. It is difficult for any instructor to be objective in assigning grades to a class of fewer than ten students, and even more so if the class is composed of fewer than five students. This evaluation is very important, however, as nearly all students receive college credit for their laboratory practicum year.

OTHER EMPLOYMENT OPPORTUNITIES

As the scope of the work in the laboratory continues to widen, employment opportunities of different kinds become available.

Although medical technologists, both male and female, are eligible for commissions in the armed forces, there are few such commissions available and the competition for selection is intense. Most of the laboratory work in military installations is done by enlisted personnel; therefore, the requirements for laboratory officers may be limited to as few as one per installation. Persistence in application for commission, plus a willingness to accept one in any branch of the armed forces, may yield results. The technologist who truly desires to obtain a commission in military service must remember that all negotiations involved in seeking a commission are conducted with recruiting office personnel of the particular branch of service. These recruiters are extremely highly motivated career military personnel and are much more receptive to persons who approach them with the question, "What can I do for my country?" and *not* "What kind of benefits do you have to bid for my talents?"

Military salaries are comparable to or exceed those for civilian positions, and military life offers many other inducements. Officers of the medical department of the armed forces and Public Health Service carry equal rank and privileges with other military officers. A military commission provides a unique opportunity for a technologist to develop and use qualities of leadership and management skills. Most technologists who receive commissions first undergo a brief period of military orientation and then assume their first permanent duty station at a military hospital. In many cases this assignment is as a Laboratory Officer or similar administrative post. As most of the routine daily laboratory workload is done by enlisted technicians, the officer's role is that of supervisor, manager, or perhaps special projects and research director. A career officer in the military service

78

may, with diligence and motivation, become the commanding officer of a military health care facility or base.

It should be realized that military officers receive changes of station periodically. Periods of duty in the continental United States may be interspersed with shorter tours of overseas duty, and often the officer may be accompanied by his dependents. This aspect of military life is generally considered one of the most attractive features of a career in the military medical department. Separations from one's family are infrequent and usually are of relatively short duration. Military retirement, which is optional after 20 years of service, is generally financially superior to most civilian retirement plans, and permits a second career without loss of military retirement pay and benefits.

Many critics of military life decry the loss of individuality that seems to be a part of entry into any government service. This is not necessarily true of the medical technologist who accepts a military commission. As a small segment of the military population, technologist/officers have access to counterpart officers in Washington and frequently are able to express their desires for future changes of duty stations. Medical department officers who remain as career military officers develop a wide range of acquaintances and friends in their service, often on a worldwide basis. The esprit de corps in the medical departments is often unknown in other areas of military life. There is also a great deal of satisfaction in working in military hospitals, for the patient population is young and resilient and the majority of patients recover from their illnesses and injuries.

The National Institutes of Health in Bethesda, Maryland, offer employment to many technologists in many fields, as does the National Center for Disease Control in Chamblee, Georgia. Equipment manufacturers employ technologists to teach the purchasers of the equipment how to use it, how to keep it in working order, and how to make small needed repairs.

Veterinary medicine offers numerous opportunities, both in research and in the veterinarian's office. It goes without saying that the technologist must have a certain affinity for animals.

There are increasing numbers of opportunities for employment abroad. Several middle eastern oil-producing nations are intensively developing health care systems and educational programs. In addition, opportunities for professional laboratory personnel and allied health educators have been developing in both Australia and New Zealand. There are few jobs on the European continent unless the person seeking one is fluent in another language besides English.

Although the Project Hope hospital ship is no longer operated,

Hope recruits medical technologists and educators for its land-based facilities. Project Hope expects to extend health programs to areas of need wherever they may be identified in the world. In this country Project Hope's first domestic program developed a curriculum at Laredo Junior College (Texas) whereby the student qualifies as a laboratory aide after the completion of the first semester, as a certified laboratory assistant at the end of the first year, and as a medical laboratory technician at the conclusion of two years of study.

Occasionally an unusual position is available, perhaps in Guam or Pago Pago. Or, the opportunity to contribute in a very real way to the betterment of mankind will arise. For example, a dermatologist organized Holidays for Humanity,[3] which arranged for medical teams, including technologists, to spend vacations in Central or South America or on a Caribbean island ministering to back-country inhabitants.

SALARIES

Numerous national and state salary surveys have been conducted in recent years, with the goal of determining identifiable trends relative to earnings of medical technologists. These surveys seem to become obsolete almost before they are published, and are therefore not included here. It is known that salaries earned by medical technologists vary widely from urban to rural areas, from small towns to large cities, and from college communities to industrial centers. The law of supply and demand heavily influences the salaries offered in many localities and institutions. Fringe benefits, security, working conditions, and advancement opportunities, not shown in salary figures, frequently obscure the significance of salary survey findings. Students seeking authoritative salary information about any particular locality or institution are encouraged to initiate inquiries with the help of their faculty advisors or local hospitals in making personal contacts.

A 1974 survey by the ASMT indicated several trends and factors that relate to salaries and that appear to be fairly typical. More administrative and chief technologists have fringe benefits entirely paid by employers than do staff technologists. More have life insurance and retirement plans. More receive reimbursement for continuing education programs. Males generally receive higher salaries than do females for equivalent positions.

The ASMT survey also described the typical medical technologist as female, between 25 and 29 years of age, with a baccalaureate degree, working as a staff technologist in a hospital of 500 or more beds. This typical technologist receives time and a half for overtime, and her fringe benefits include vacation, holidays, sick leave and medical insurance, the latter partially paid by her employer.

THE FUTURE OF MEDICAL TECHNOLOGY

It should now be obvious that medical technology offers many opportunities in a wide variety of positions. It also offers both lateral and vertical mobility—lateral with variety in the kinds of positions and vertical in terms of responsibility.

To attempt to picture with clarity and accuracy the characteristics of the laboratory of the future is almost sheer folly. However, certain apparently well-defined trends can be discerned. One of these, the increase in the numbers of commercially owned and operated laboratories, has already been mentioned.

The university medical center laboratory will continue its present functions: "To educate physicians and other health programs, to conduct research into basic problems of disease, and to evaluate better methods of diagnosis and treatment."[4]

The trend towards automation and computerization has had the general effect of reducing the versatility of small laboratories. The general effect has been toward the establishment of central or regional laboratories. A concomitant improvement in transportation facilities must be assumed. The installation on which the centralization of laboratory services will no doubt have the greatest effect will be the small community hospital laboratory. About 50 percent of all hospitals registered by the American Hospital Association have fewer than 250 beds. Many small hospitals, particularly those in rural areas, have difficulty in attracting pathologists and medical technologists. A satellite laboratory in each of these installations, supervised by a visiting pathologist or a clinical laboratory scientist and staffed by persons trained in a minimum number of procedures, could provide emergency service, with all other procedures being referred to the central laboratory.

Increased numbers of people having hospital insurance coverage or participating in the Medicare program, the introduction of multiphasic screening of people of all ages, and the continued participation of the government in sponsored research will all influence the spiraling demands for laboratory work and medical technologists. It does not seem overly optimistic to predict that the future of medical technology will be bright, although the kinds of positions and the work done may be different.

Manpower needs will necessarily change to reflect the increase in automated procedures. Students often express a fear that automation will phase out medical technologists, since it is not necessary to have a college education in order to learn how to push buttons. With the rapid technological changes we see today it is impossible to predict with certainty how future developments will affect the profession. It is quite possible that medical technologists will become specialists in single areas, working as supervisors. Preparation for such a position might well include experience in depth in one area plus concentration on instruction in, and development of, managerial skills.

If the staffing patterns in an automated and computerized laboratory are viewed as a pyramid, the base will represent those workers required to maintain, repair, and operate the instrumentation of the laboratory. The second stratum will encompass a large group of workers capable of doing those procedures not automated, or maintaining reagents, and preparing blood components. These workers may include those with training equivalent to the present medical laboratory technician and the baccalaureate level medical technologist. The third group will be medical technologists with training in depth in one area (specialists), probably all with masters' degrees. They would function as section supervisors, maintaining quality control programs, devising and testing new procedures, and supervising subordinate personnel. At the apex will be the clinical laboratory scientist with the doctoral degree. He will have general supervision of all areas. He will act in conjunction with the pathologist or may supplant him in institutions not having a pathologist in residence.

Perhaps a look at the manpower needs for the future will show the reasons for the optimistic employment outlook. Countless surveys of manpower needs have been conducted over the years. Often these surveys had little or no relevance to the actual problem, since a favorite question included in the questionnaires was "how many technologists would you hire if adequately trained persons were available?" The answer often indicated an ideal situation that had little or no resemblance to the actual economic possibilities. Distinguishing between a desirable or ideal level of personnel requirements and the actual shortage of laboratory workers often changes the figures.

A significant factor in the laboratory manpower situation, both present and future, is the enactment of the Clinical Laboratory Improvement Act of 1976. This federal legislation sets minimum personnel standards for nearly all laboratories which receive funds from federal sources in payment for laboratory services.

The Manpower Administration of the United States Department of Labor prepared a report of *Technology and Manpower in the*

Health Service Industry, 1965–1975.[4] The base estimate for 1965 indicates approximately 100,000 laboratory workers were employed, about 80 percent in hospitals, the other 20 percent in private offices, private laboratories, etc. An additional 27,000 were estimated to be working outside the health service industry. The figures were broken down as follows:

Medical technologists, technicians, and scientists 60,000
Laboratory assistants 25,000
Laboratory helpers, orderlies, etc. 15,000

The estimate for 1975 includes a 40 percent increase in the number of workers listed above (160,000) and an increase of 16,000 workers outside the health service industry, for a grand total of 203,000. These figures were based "partly on statistical evidence, partly on factual data, somewhat on subjective judgments."[4] Spence and Bering,[5] in assembling clinical laboratory manpower data, estimated that approximately 170,000 personnel held some type of certification in 1976.

One of the best summaries of needs is that based on the workload of the laboratory. Such a summary is found in *Manpower for the Medical Laboratory*.[6]

Predictions of laboratory workloads usually start with a base of at least a half-billion clinical diagnostic tests performed in 1966. Projections that this will double by 1975 to at least a billion have been called conservative. The workload in clinical chemistry laboratories has doubled approximately every five years during the past two decades (average increase in tests of 15 per cent per year), and this rate of growth is expected to continue.

In the next 10-15 years, automation is expected to triple or quadruple the capacity of laboratories in general hospitals. However, while automation will bring about increased efficiency per technician hour, most observers agree that these gains usually are offset by requests for a larger quantity of work, resulting in increases in manpower needs.

... what is obvious is that more manpower is needed now and will be needed in the future, more hands with better education and better training, capable of fulfilling a variety of vital tasks in a variety of settings, all aimed at the fundamental goal of helping the diagnostic team find the hidden causes and cures of diseases.

The next decade promises to be the most exciting and challenging period in the development of laboratory medicine. Medical technologists are sometimes hesitant to contemplate the inevitability of change. Yet those who can look back over the years before World War II realize the immensities of the changes and the progress which resulted. Change began with the establishment of the laboratory, and innovation is merely the expected direction of what must be an unrelenting drive toward continual improvement of laboratory service and patient care. Change should not threaten any prospective student, but rather should be viewed as an instrument by which the continual improvement may be accomplished.

REFERENCES

1. U. S. Civil Service Commission: *Working for the U. S. A.* Pamphlet 4, April, 1969.

2. Industry sends technologist training team into field. Lab. World *21:*75, 1970.

3. Cross, Wilbur: How to get more out of your vacation. Reader's Digest *97(3):*113-116, 1970.

4. Sturm, Herman M.: *Technology and Manpower in the Health Service Industry.* Manpower Administration, U. S. Dept. of Labor, 1966.

5. Spence, H. A. and Bering, N. M.: Credentialing in the clinical laboratories. Am. J. Med. Technol. *44:*393-397, 1978.

6. *Manpower for the Medical Laboratory.* Proceedings of a Conference of Government and the Professions. 1967.

SUGGESTED READINGS

Educational qualifications of public health laboratory workers. Public Health *57:*523-531, 1967.

Kinney, Thomas D., and Robert S. Melville: The clinical laboratory scientist. Lab. Invest. *20:*382-389, 1969.

Part II is titled "Structure and function of clinical laboratories of the future." It describes the functions of the regional medical laboratory, the university center laboratory, the community hospital laboratory, and the independent laboratory.

Part III, "The clinical laboratory scientist of the future," describes the four areas in which laboratory scientists will work—basic research, applied research and development, laboratory management, and laboratory service. The qualifications that may be required for each area are outlined.

LaCroix, K. A.: An examination of the expanded role for medical technologists. Am. J. Med. Technol. *44:*373-376, 1978.

Lucas, Fred, Thomas L. Lincoln, and Thomas D. Kinney: Clinical laboratory science. Lab. Invest. *20:*400-404, 1969. The subtitle of the article, "A look to the future," is indicative of the contents.

McCrimmon, Aubry: The medical technologist in industry. Cadence *2:*25, 1971.

New directions for MT mobility. MLO *4:*(May-June) 1972. The entire issue is devoted to descriptions of different kinds of positions.

Oliver, R. E.: Job satisfaction in medical technology. Lab. Med. *9:*30-32, 58, 1978.

Roach, Gregory: Unionization and the professional. Cadence *4:*39-42, 1973.

Unionization: pro and con. MLO (special issue) *6:*(Spring) 1974. The entire issue is devoted to the pros and cons of the trend toward unionization in the laboratory.

8

Professional Ethics

Ethics is defined as principles of conduct governing an individual or a group.* Usually a profession includes among its distinguishing characteristics a provision for self-regulation and a code of ethics. Most of the health-related professions, including medical technology, have such codes.

CODE OF ETHICS

A discussion of the Code of Ethics is considered pertinent to the study of medical technology for these reasons:

1. Every student entering medical technology should be sufficiently interested in the profession to support it by membership in the society that represents him. As a member he should be aware of the existence of a Code of Ethics that dictates his actions as a professional.
2. The development of the Code of Ethics demonstrates a phase in the maturation of the organization.

When the proposal for a Registry of Laboratory Technicians was

---

* *Webster's New Collegiate Dictionary*. Springfield, Massachusetts, G. and C. Merriam Company, 1973.

submitted to the American Society of Clinical Pathologists, it contained a statement of a code of ethics that those who were registered would agree to follow.

> All registered technicians and technologists shall be required to strictly observe the Code of Ethics as defined by the American Society of Clinical Pathologists, namely, that they shall agree to work at all times under the supervision of a qualified physician and shall under no circumstances, on their own initiative, render written or oral diagnoses except insofar as it is self-evident in the report, or advise physicians or others in the treatment of disease, or operate a laboratory independently without the supervision of a qualified physician or clinical pathologist.[1]

When the bylaws of the newly organized American Society of Medical Technologists (ASMT) were written, Article VIII, Section 1 stated: "The Code of Ethics of this society shall be the same as that prescribed by the Registry of Technicians of the American Society of Clinical Pathologists." It is obvious, however, that the society was not entirely satisfied with the status quo, since the subject was discussed at the 1941 convention. The delegates voted to retain the Code of Ethics as "put out by the Registry."

In 1947 an amendment to the bylaws was adopted which read: "This association may adopt a Code of Ethics which shall govern the professional conduct of the active members." At the same time the delegates did not exercise the right or privilege they had just incorporated into the bylaws and accepted the resolution of the Board of Directors that the Board of Registry retain "the present code of ethics" and "interpret it literally."

At the 1949 convention another code was presented. One section was rejected by the delegates. It read: "Nothing in this Code of Ethics shall be inconsistent with that of the American Society of Clinical Pathologists and that of the American Medical Association." This may have been the first successful effort to acknowledge that the society could exist separate from the Registry and the American Society of Clinical Pathologists.

The Code of Ethics published in the 1955 bylaws read:

> Section 1. A member of this Society shall at all times work only under the direction and supervision of a pathologist or duly qualified doctor of medicine or specialist in one of the divisions of clinical pathology, such qualifications being determined on the basis of accepted medical ethics.
>
> Section 2. A member of this Society shall make no diagnosis or interpretations other than those in the reports prepared by him.
>
> Section 3. A member of this Society shall not advise physicians or others how to treat disease.

Section 4.   A member of this Society shall not train students without supervision of a clinical pathologist.

Section 5.   A member of this Society shall not engage in laboratory work independent of qualified supervision (as provided in Section 1) nor shall he operate an independent laboratory.

Section 6.   It is ethical to perform laboratory work on a commission basis under contract with a public health, research, or clinical laboratory when such work is done as provided in Section 1 above and when all contractual agreements are approved and signed by the director of the organization contracting for such services.

With the exceptions of Sections 4 and 6 this code is merely a somewhat longer version of the original one incorporated in the Registry proposal. Section 4 was added to the Registry code when it was required that all students certified by the Registry should have had their clinical experiences in an approved school. The present Code of Ethics was adopted in 1957.

> Being fully cognizant of my responsibilities in the practice of Medical Technology, I affirm my willingness to discharge my duties with accuracy, thoughtfulness, and care.
>
> Realizing that the knowledge obtained concerning patients in the course of my work must be treated as confidential I hold inviolate the confidence (trust) placed in me by patient and physician.
>
> Recognizing that my integrity and that of my profession must be pledged to the absolute reliability of my work, I will conduct myself at all times in a manner appropriate to the dignity of my profession.

A short time later the same code appeared in the literature of the Registry, with the previous code incorporated in Standards of Conduct. There had been one addition to the first section to cover the expansion of work into laboratories other than those in hospitals or doctors' offices. "It is ethical to work as a medical technologist in a research laboratory, a Public Health Laboratory or accredited teaching institution when such work is done under the direction or supervision of a duly qualified doctor of medicine."

Each yearly edition of the booklet, *The Registry of Medical Technologists of the American Society of Clinical Pathologists*, contained both the code and the sections on conduct until that published in 1970 when both were eliminated. This elimination occurred because of investigation by the Justice Department which found sections 1, 2, and 6 unnecessarily restrictive and monopolistic.

The Code of Ethics appeared on the reverse side of the membership card with a place for the member's signature below it. Objections were raised by some members, but the signature line has remained.

The enforcement of the Code of Ethics is now the sole responsibility of the ASMT. Since the code is formulated and enforced by peers, the organization now fulfills another of the basic requirements of a profession.

A STUDENT CODE OF ETHICS

Student medical technologists likewise should be guided by a code of ethics. The author's students were asked to develop a code of ethics that they felt would express their responsibilities in the areas of personal conduct and their relationship to the medical staff and to the patients. It was requested that the code be realistic enough to be followed and definitive enough that other students would understand their responsibilities. The following code was developed with only minor assistance from the instructors.

CODE OF ETHICS FOR STUDENT MEDICAL TECHNOLOGISTS
Developed at the University of Florida by the Class of 1967

We, as students of Medical Technology, will apply the following code of ethics to our actions toward patients, physicians, and hospital personnel in our clinical year of training and in our future work. This code will apply to our personal as well as professional attitudes and conduct.

As PROFESSIONALS we will:

1. Assume a professional manner in attire and conduct
2. Establish a rapport with hospital staff, supervisors, and physicians
3. Hold in confidence information relating to patients
4. Strive for increased efficiency and quality through organization
5. Be willing to accept responsibility for our own work and results
6. Strive to learn the theories of laboratory determinations
7. Establish confidence of the patient through kindness and empathy

In PERSONAL conduct we will:

1. Achieve the highest degree of honesty and integrity
2. Maintain adaptability in action and attitude
3. Establish a sense of fraternity among fellow students
4. Strive to have a pleasant manner in the laboratory and with the patients
5. Remember that we are University as well as Medical Technology students; therefore we should strive to be educated individuals outside our technical field.

Almost every student will find at least one facet or phase of his clinical laboratory experience difficult, annoying, or downright discouraging. How one student managed to overcome the problems she encountered is described in a paper she wrote near the end of her year in the clinical laboratory.

HOW TO SUCCEED AT BEING A MEDICAL TECHNOLOGY STUDENT
Janet Anne McChesney Jetton*

The question most often asked of medical technology students about to enter their year of training is, "What is it like?" Very often, the answer to that question does not present itself until the year is nearly finished. This paper, written by a student just completing that year, is an attempt to set forth a few guideposts for the neophyte medical technologist.

Let us begin with that nebulous quality so popular on student evaluation sheets—attitude. What is attitude? Webster defines it as "position or bearing as indicating action, feeling, or mood . . . hence, the feeling or mood itself . . ." I define attitude as the most important aspect not only of your 12-months' training period, but also of your entire career as a medical technologist.

You say, "Isn't it just a bit more important to have technical skill and knowledge of what you are doing?" My answer to that is another question, "How can you possibly achieve technical excellence if you have no motivation?" Your attitude is your motivating force. It is because you care about what you are doing and why you are doing it that you do something well.

Because you chose this profession in the first place, I assume that you have a basic interest in it. This basic interest forms the foundation of your attitude. With this basic interest comes enthusiasm, which is invaluable to you. True, your enthusiasm may wane at times, but if securely rooted, it will always come back and get you through the doldrums.

Another important part of your attitude is your willingness to follow instruction and to accept criticism, your willingness to work and to study. You should be happy with your work and take pride in it. You should take pride in your profession as a whole. *You* chose it, so it must be good!

As part of your attitude, develop a professional air. What is a professional air, or concept? Well, it certainly is not a severe hairdo, horn-rimmed glasses, and use of words a layman cannot comprehend. A professional air is that dignity and pride which comes from knowing that the work you are doing is important work. It is understanding your work and the ability to discuss it intelligently, in technical terms with your colleagues, but also in terms intelligible to laymen. It is your sense of duty, the serious purpose with which you do your work. It is diligence, courtesy, competence, and respect.

Attitude is mainly caring—caring about your profession, your work, and about getting along with all of the people you come in contact with in the course of your work.

During your rotation as a student, you will find there are laboratories which you will like more than others. This is perfectly all right. If everyone liked only microbiology, what would we do for blood bank technologists? But, bear in mind the fact that each lab, in the final analysis, is exactly what you make it. If there is one which you think you are really going to hate, make a special effort to really like that lab. Try a little harder there—you may come out of that department truly liking it. I know; it happened to me! As a student, I made it a point to enter each department of the laboratories with an open mind and a charitable heart. It works wonders, really.

Next comes responsibility. I have heard so many times, "How do you teach responsibility?" It is my belief that responsibility is neither taught nor learned.

---

* Graduated from University of Florida, 1965. Reproduced by permission.

Responsibility is given and responsibility is accepted. When you decide to become a medical technologist, you are aware of the great responsibility you must accept. Any error, carelessness, or incompetence on your part can be costly to the patient and/or to yourself.

When you apply to a training program, you are stating your willingness to accept this responsibility. When you are accepted in a training program, those in charge are stating their willingness to extend this responsibility to you. Your actions from then on are the mark of whether you have "learned" responsibility.

Let us now discuss in more detail some of your more specific responsibilities as a medical technologist. Your first responsibility is to the patient (if you do not care about him, what are you doing in this profession?). Your second responsibility is a dual one: first, to your pathologist and house staff (after all, your profession was founded as an aid to them); and second, to your fellow workers (a clinical laboratory is a taut ship and requires above all, cooperation).

Your contact with the patient will depend on the type and size of your laboratory. Some medical technologists have little or no contact with the patient personally. Still, you must remember that the results of the tests you perform are going to directly affect him. If you do have direct contact with the patient, there are several things you should bear in mind. First of all, remember that the things you have to do to him are not pleasant; and secondly, remember that he is a patient because he is ill and when people do not feel well, they are, with a few exceptions, not exactly jolly. You must never become angry with an irritable patient. He *can't* help it; *you* can! Since you cannot make him like what you are doing (*nobody* loves a venipuncture), try to make him like *you*. Those times when you have an uncooperative patient are the times you have to remember that you are a medical technologist because you care about *him*. It is not really difficult to be pleasant and just plain nice, and it *is* possible to make those few minutes you spend with the patient a bright spot in his day.

The next of your responsibilities is that to your pathologist and house staff. The tests you perform are diagnostic tests for the physician. You are invaluable to him, even though he sometimes may forget that. We have heard many stories about friction between the laboratory personnel and the physician. He may expect results before you have had time to complete the test, or he may question you if the results of a test are not consistent with his presumptive diagnosis. Once again rises the need for a little kindness and understanding. His main concern is for his patient, as is yours. Therefore, you must be a team, not antagonists. Work for and with your pathologist and physician, not against them. Kindness and cooperation are contagious.

Now, your most immediate responsibility—that to your fellow workers. This is where cooperation really counts. Everyone in a laboratory must be efficient and accurate. There is no room for error. Inasmuch as this in itself creates a tension situation, there is, therefore, no room in a clinical laboratory for personal conflict or childish behavior. Each of us has his own set of personal characteristics, some of which can be quite irritating to others. Most laboratories provide close working quarters. This can be conducive to getting the work done efficiently, but it can also be conducive to personality conflicts. Here is a place where your good attitude can be put to use. If you are conscientious and interested in your work, aware of the need for accuracy and efficiency, you will also be aware of the dangers of personal friction. No one can do his best when under an emotional strain, and a medical technologist must *always* do his best.

As long as people remain human and as long as each personality remains a separate entity, occasions of conflict will arise. That is why it is so very important for all laboratory personnel to consciously try to avoid it. Each member of the laboratory team must have respect for the other's ability. As a student, your position will be a rather precarious one. You will be given a job to do, you will be expected to do it well, and you will be under constant observation.

Since no one pops out of the mold with "Medical Technologist" stamped across his back, an AutoAnalyzer for a brain, and his fingertips tingling with skill, you will probably be slow and rather awkward at first. This is one of those times to pick yourself up by your good attitude and keep plugging away until you do acquire the necessary skills. When you are corrected or criticized constructively, be grateful. Practice of a good habit makes perfect; practice of a bad habit makes poor technique which is very difficult to unlearn. Remember that it is much better to ask a question and appear a little stupid, than to make a mistake which may lead to an erroneous report which can possibly endanger the patient.

Keep your wits about you at all times; you can learn something from everyone. Maintain your enthusiasm, but at the same time be quiet and attentive. Try to be pleasant with everyone. All of us have our bad days, and the staff members can sometimes be rather short with a student. You can avoid this with a little diplomacy. If and when this happens, remember that you *are* a student and keep your respect for your superiors. They already have what you are working so hard for, so they deserve your respect. Very rare, indeed, is the person who will not help you if you ask him sincerely and if you are willing to work. And work you will! And acquire excellence you will—if you work and try and try and try again.

Because ours is such a dynamic and ever-changing field, a medical technologist never stops learning. Each of us should consider it a moral obligation to teach each new thing we learn to someone else. And always, always, be charitable—to the patient, to the physician, to your superiors, to your fellow workers, and when the time comes, to *your* students.

In conclusion, I would like to insert my favorite little prayer, a few words which helped me over the rough spots of my training:

God grant me the serenity to accept the things I cannot change, the courage
to change the things I can, the wisdom to know the difference.

REFERENCES

1. Report of Committee to ASCP. J. Lab. Clin. Med. *14*:493, 1929.

The references to the various codes of ethics have been excerpted from printed bylaws of the ASMT.

9

Professional Organizations and Registries

An organization of persons with similar professional interests is, or should be, a clearly representative voice of those persons. Its purpose is to increase the recognition and the prestige of the group. It represents the profession to the public, before government agencies, and to other professional organizations. Every medical technologist should be interested enough in his profession to join the professional organization that represents him. His support of the organization gives him a feeling of participation in the enhancement of the stature and status of his profession. It also enables him to add his voice to those of his peers, for greater effect.

PROFESSIONAL ORGANIZATIONS

American Society of Clinical Pathologists

The American Society of Clinical Pathologists (ASCP) is the professional organization devoted to the interests of those engaged in the medical specialty of pathology and to the encouragement of research in the clinical laboratory. Seven classes of membership are offered. Full membership, called a fellowship, is granted to pathologists who have been certified by the American Board of Pathology. Junior membership is open to physicians who have completed two years of specialty training in pathology. Physicians and nonphysician scientists may become associate members. There are also Honorary and Emeritus fellows and foreign members. Persons who have been certified in one of the technical categories as designated by the ASCP may become affiliate members. This latter type of membership is open to registered medical technologists, as well as to others.

The first opportunity to join ASCP as an affiliate member came in 1969, shortly after the American Society for Medical Technology filed a suit against ASCP. The stated reasons for opening membership were: "To establish better and closer channels of communication with medical technologists certified by the Board of Registry, and to broaden opportunities for their participation in ASCP continuing education programs and their utilization of education materials developing from these programs."[1]

ASCP, in a rather extensive educational program, offers a number of workshops, seminars, and scientific meetings to pathologists and medical technologists at many locations and times throughout each year. These offerings, plus ASCP's full catalog of educational materials and publications, are offered to affiliate members, usually at a discount.

ASCP's services and offerings directed toward non-pathologist medical laboratory personnel have greatly increased in the late 1970s. Notable among these is the significant reduction in fees charged these personnel for continuing education offerings, and a system to acknowledge their participation in professional continuing education.

The American Society for Medical Technology (ASMT) in 1969 opposed membership for medical technologists in ASCP, contending that this offer of membership was "a disguised effort to maintain control of the medical laboratory personnel at a time when other monopolistic activities in the medical laboratory have been declared illegal."[2] ASCP disagreed with this contention, which became one aspect of litigation later initiated by ASMT.

College of American Pathologists

The College of American Pathologists (CAP) is the outgrowth of the separation of the educational, research, and socioeconomic activities from the scientific and business portions of the ASCP. To be eligible for full membership, a physician must be a diplomate of the American Board of Pathology. About 80 percent of the physicians who are members of the ASCP also belong to CAP.

American Society for Medical Technology

The American Society of Clinical Laboratory Technicians was

93

organized in 1933 and held its first national convention that year. The name was changed to the American Society of Medical Technologists (ASMT) in 1936, and again changed in 1972 to the American Society for Medical Technology.

The Society is dedicated to:

1. Establishing, developing, and maintaining the highest standards in clinical laboratory methods and research;
2. Creating mutual understanding and cooperation between those in the laboratory and all health professionals working in the interest of individual and public health;
3. Promoting programs of primary and continuing education, research, and development;
4. Representing the profession of medical technology through improvement of the status of its members;
5. Advancing the ideals and principles of the profession of medical technology.[3]

The definitions of membership requirements have been subject to much debate at ASMT annual meetings, to the extent that at the 1974 meeting it was decided that no membership qualifications would be changed for at least two years. Discussion continues unabated, and nearly every year some changes are made in membership qualifications. In 1978, an ASMT membership application gave the following qualifications for active membership:

Baccalaureate/graduate degree in medical technology or related science; OR License and certification from an agency recognized by ASMT and in an area of laboratory science; OR five years experience in medical laboratory science; OR completed attendance at an accredited structured program of training in medical laboratory science.

Application for membership in the ASMT must be made in conjunction with an application for membership in a constituent society (state or District of Columbia). In other words, it is not possible to maintain membership solely in a constituent society, nor is it possible to be a member of only the national Society, except for corresponding members.

The House of Delegates is the governing body of the Society. Its membership consists of the president and president-elect of each constituent society, the delegates designated by each constituent society, and the members of the Board of Directors.[4]

The number of delegates to which each constituent society is entitled is determined by the number of members in that society at the close of the fiscal year of the ASMT (April 30). The number of delegates in excess of the president and president-elect is based upon a formula of one delegate for each 50 active members or major portion thereof. In addition, each constituent society is entitled to one voting student delegate in the House, regardless of the number of student members affiliated with that constituent society.[4]

The House of Delegates convenes at the annual meeting. It meets twice during each session. The first meeting is that of the Presidents Council, comprised of the president and president-elect of each constituent society, the national officers and the Board of Directors. The second meeting is the full House of Delegates, traditionally conducted near the end of the annual session. The Board of Directors represents the Society between meetings of the House of Delegates. The Board is comprised of the national officers, the immediate past president, and one regional director from each of ten designated geographic areas.

The accomplishments of the ASMT have been numerous and far-reaching. The membership has grown from an ineffective group of about 500 in 1937 to a 1978 strength of over 30,000. The Society speaks strongly for the profession.

Two other major milestones in the Society's accomplishments are deserving of further mention. In cooperation with Central Michigan University, ASMT has established a graduate degree program tailored to meet the needs of the employed technologist. The courses are all offered in an off-campus format, in the form of workshops and seminars. It is possible for enrollees to earn either a Master of Arts in Management and Supervision or a Master of Arts in Education. The courses are generally two to four days in duration and are often available in conjunction with state, regional, or national ASMT meetings. Many other offerings are presented in numerous cities across the country and on a variety of dates.

Another major educational program offered by ASMT is that of recording the continuing education activities of ASMT members and other laboratorians who desire to enroll in the recording program. Titled *Professional Acknowledgment for Continuing Education* (P.A.C.E.), this ASMT service offers participants an annual "transcript" that lists all continuing education activities attended and courses completed.

A unique feature of the P.A.C.E. program is that a program approval request must be submitted to ASMT for review, providing such information as detailed descriptions of educational objectives, methods for evaluation, and other data that will assist the P.A.C.E. program committee to determine that a worthwhile and well-organized program is proposed. Programs that fall short of desired levels of quality are offered assistance in planning and revising their offerings so as to afford participants maximum program quality. In this way, ASMT stimulates educational providers to present only quality educational experiences to P.A.C.E. participants. This program has become a popular membership service offered by ASMT. It is also available to nonmembers for a nominal charge.

Other membership services offered by the American Society for Medical Technology include a comprehensive insurance program. Members of ASMT may obtain reasonably priced group insurance policies for Life Insurance, Hospital Cash, Hospital Income Insurance, Accidental Death and Dismemberment, Cancer Coverage and Professional Liability Insurance for both members and student members.

The American Society for Medical Technology has earned national recognition for its promotion of professionalism and for its enhancement of the stature of the medical technologist as a member of the health care team. These latter accomplishments are perhaps the most significant and noteworthy, and deserving of the appreciation of members and nonmembers alike.

During 1968 and 1969 the relations between the ASMT and the ASCP became somewhat less than amicable. The presidents of ASMT for these and succeeding years provided many communications to keep the membership informed of progress, or lack of it, in the attempts to mediate the problems.

The initial problems arose because of general discontent (on the part of ASMT members) with the management of affairs of the Board of Registry. It was the contention of ASMT that medical technologists were afforded no real voice in the determination of their own certification process. The breach opened in this dispute further widened when the ASCP established the Medical Laboratory Technician as a third category of laboratory worker (in addition to the previously established MT and CLA categories), without consulting the Board of Registry. Communications between the two societies deteriorated until, in May, 1969, the ASMT filed a suit against ASCP in the United States District Court of the Northern District of Illinois. The suit consisted of a number of specific complaints which primarily related to a perceived domination of the clinical laboratory professions by ASCP.[5]

The lawsuit caused much comment, both favorable and unfavorable, in the clinical laboratory community. It did, however, bring the attention of the laboratory professions to the roles that various professionals fill in the delivery of quality health care. A summary judgment was rendered in March, 1971, that ASMT had no cause for action. The judgment was appealed, but later the suit was dropped.

Subsequent to the termination of the legal confrontation, a period of cooperation developed in the relationship between the two societies. As previously mentioned, they have cooperated in phasing out the old Board of Schools in favor of the new jointly founded National Accrediting Agency for Clinical Laboratory Sciences. Although many old scars from "the lawsuit" remain, clear heads have sometimes prevailed in the ensuing years. Relationships again deteriorated in the late 1970s, as ASMT leaders established, with financial support from ASMT, a new "independent" certification agency for laboratory personnel. This is further discussed in Chapter 10. This action created a situation in which two professional registries are competing to examine the same population of newly-graduating students.

American Society for Microbiology

The requirement for membership in the American Society for Microbiology is a bachelor's degree in microbiology or a related field, or its equivalent in training and experience.

American Medical Technologists

American Medical Technologists (AMT) is a registry certifying medical technologists, medical laboratory technicians, and medical assistants. Founded in 1939 as a member-owned and -operated national registry for clinical laboratory personnel, it has grown to an active membership in excess of 13,000 in 1978. Since its inception AMT has certified in excess of 30,000 laboratory workers. The Accrediting Bureau of Health Education Schools, Elkhart, Indiana, an independent agency of AMT, is on the USOE list of recognized accrediting agencies. Certification by AMT is contingent upon meeting academic/experience standards and either passing a registry examination administered by AMT, or an equivalent examination acceptable to the Registry.

The requirements for eligibility for AMT registry examinations are:

MEDICAL TECHNOLOGIST. The candidate must have at least a bachelor's degree in medical technology or a bachelor's degree with a major in one of the biological sciences plus at least one year of approved laboratory experience, *or* at least three years (90 credit hours) of courses including at least 40 credit hours in the sciences to include at least 12 in chemistry, 12 in bacteriology and/or parasitology, 6 in mathematics and 8 in one of several specified biological sciences, plus one year of approved laboratory experience, *or* in the case of graduates of military or professional schools, shall have met the re-

97

quirements for Medical Laboratory Technician (AMT) and have three years of experience. MLT's (AMT) with three years of additional approved latoratory experience are also eligible to write the MT certification exam.

In addition, AMT may, upon review of credentials, register persons who have graduated from an AMT-approved school prior to November 1965 and who have four years of experience, and who pass the AMT certifying exam for MT's.

Persons not otherwise qualified for AMT certification but who have passed the HEW Proficiency Exam will be permitted to take the AMT certification examination for MT's.

Applicants who meet AMT training and experience requirements may be registered by AMT if they present evidence of holding other certifications by examinations that are acceptable to the AMT Board of Directors.

MEDICAL LABORATORY TECHNICIAN. All applicants for certification by AMT as an MLT must meet one of the following requirements:

Completion of at least two years (60 semester hours) of courses in an accredited college or community college, including 12 hours in chemistry, bacteriology, parasitology, in any combination; three hours in mathematics, eight hours in several areas of the biological sciences, plus six months of approved laboratory experience, *or*

completion of an Associate of Science degree in medical technology (or equivalent) from an accredited junior college, with six months of additional approved laboratory experience, *or*

graduation from a medical laboratory school accredited by the Accrediting Bureau of Health Education Schools (18 months course followed by six months approved experience, or 12 months school and 12 months experience); *or*

completion of a course of at least 50 weeks duration in a U.S. Armed Forces school of medical technology, followed by approved laboratory experience to provide a total of education and experience equivalent to the requirements given above. All of the above must pass the AMT/MLT examination.

Applicants holding other certifications by examinations in the MLT category may be considered for registration without further examination[7] providing the applicants meet AMT training/experience standards.

The American Medical Technologists publish the *Journal of the American Medical Technologists*, which contains scientific papers,

Registry (Society) news, legislative and industry reports, book reviews, and editoral content.

In recent years, AMT and ASMT have established working communications with each other. There are now a number of states and regions where joint conventions are held and where state and local groups of the two organizations meet regularly and cooperate fully in considering mutual concerns. In Florida, for example, the state societies of AMT and ASMT have joined with the Florida Society of Medical Technologists, an independent group, in sponsoring joint spring conventions. Each year one of the organizations serves as host society, and an agreement has been reached for sharing the convention proceeds among all three. The three organizations in Florida have also joined with a number of other laboratory-oriented groups to jointly sponsor a non-profit educational foundation dedicated to continuing education for laboratory personnel in that state.

International Association of Medical Laboratory Technologists

As the name implies, the International Association of Medical Laboratory Technologists (IAMLT) is an organization to provide communication among the technologists of different countries. The association hosts an annual convention to which ASMT sends delegates. Membership is not open to individuals but to organizations. The ASMT is an organizational member.

International Society of Clinical Laboratory Technology

The International Society of Clinical Laboratory Technology is not to be confused with the IAMLT. The ISCLT sponsors a Credentialing Commission, "an autonomous body composed of leaders in the fields of medicine, education, hospital administration and clinical laboratory services,"[8] which establishes requirements for certification by ISCLT, reviews all applications for ISCLT certification, and establishes criteria for the ISCLT's continuing education programs.

The ISCLT also provides a service for recording continuing education activities of members.

ISCLT has five general classes of members: Registrant, Regular, Student, Educational, and Sustaining. The latter four classes do not require registration as an RMT for membership.

The requirements for eligibility for examination for Registered Medical Technologist (RMT) are that an individual must have one of the following:

1. A baccalaureate degree from an accredited university or college, with a major in chemical, physical or biological science,

and a minimum of one year of acceptable clinical laboratory experience.

2. Be a Registered Laboratory Technician (RLT) with five years of experience acceptable to the Credentialing Commission and with acceptable Continuing Education Units.

3. Recognized by Medicare as a medical technologist or general supervisor.

Individuals who successfully challenge the HEW Proficiency Examination are not required to write the ISCLT examination.

The ISCLT offers many membership benefits, and the Society's publications indicate the strong support of the concept of career mobility, "vertically, institutionally, and geographically." In 1978, the Society's membership consisted of around 9,700 persons.

STUDENT INVOLVEMENT

Students in medical laboratory science should be and are interested in their chosen profession. They have been offered an opportunity to assume an active role in the American Society for Medical Technology. Some difficulties are of course inherent in the participation of students in the activities of the Society. Annual state and national conventions are usually held in June, about the time that most students have had an opportunity to learn what the laboratory and the Society are all about. Since they are then nearly at the end of their one year of practicum experience, the well-informed student delegate to a national convention will probably not be a student after the convention is over, for graduation will have taken place about the same time. However, new trends in the age and experience of student members of the Society are being seen. Many students are joining ASMT during their junior (or earlier) years, and many students in two-year MLT programs are joining when they are at the college freshman level. This tends to increase the number of students who are ASMT members for two or more years and has markedly stimulated the activity in the student arena.

Students began as nonvoting participants in ASMT in 1969, when the House of Delegates created a student section of the ASMT Scientific Assembly to provide a forum for student members. In 1973, the House of Delegates approved a bylaws change which provided that one student from each state would be a voting delegate in the House of Delegates. In 1974, students were seated for the first time in the House of Delegates, and their contributions to the business proceedings were received by the House with obvious approval and enthusiasm. The ASMT Student Forum now enjoys representation on the Board of Directors of ASMT, and provides a voice for the interests and concerns of students in Society matters.

At the 1970 ASMT national meeting, a prospectus was given to students who were in attendance, in order to guide them in the formation of a student organization. Because it clearly outlines the organization of the student section it is included here.[9]

STUDENT SECTION OF THE SCIENTIFIC ASSEMBLY PROSPECTUS

Purpose

The purpose of this section will be to develop a feeling of pride and professionalism in students of medical technology through student membership in their professional organization, ASMT.

Our goal is to improve the field of Medical Technology via an exchange of student ideas.

We wish to unite all students in order to help solve some of our common problems through:

1. Nation-wide communication between students.
2. The development and maintenance of interest in the field of Medical Technology for the recruitment and retention of Medical Technology students.
3. Exposure of Medical Technology students to their professional organization in order to create interest in ASMT and to promote membership of recent Medical Technology graduates.
4. Presentation of student problems to ASMT.
5. Encouraging continuing education through presentation of scientific papers, seminars and workshops on a national level.

Table of Organization

1. Three national officers: Chairman, vice-chairman, secretary-treasurer.
2. Three committee chairmen: Publications, nominations, membership.
3. Advisors:
   A. ASMT Liaison
   B. Previous year's officers

Although the prospectus does not outline specific goals, a fact sheet available at the same convention indicated the goals for that year were promotion of the formation of campus and state organizations and a critique of the medical technology curricula with suggestions for reform.

Students have been encouraged to form campus and state organizations, and outlines of essential factors for organization were provided in 1969 by the student assembly. These may be helpful to readers who wish to consider establishing their own student group and are included here for their information.

ESSENTIALS FOR FORMING A STUDENT ORGANIZATION ON CAMPUS

A. Interest and people

B. Stimulate interest in as large a group as possible so that actions represent a consensus of potential members

C. Objectives:

1. Student participation on student-faculty committees; e.g., curriculum committees, administrative committees, evaluation committees, etc.

2. Encourage inter-relationship of students in Medical Technology throughout their four years.

3. Develop initiative.

4. Develop relationships with students in other health science programs.

5. Develop social/educational activities.

6. Promotion of Medical Technology in general.

D. Bylaws

E. Money

F. Advisors

G. Affiliation with campus student government.

1. Meaningful voice in campus affairs.

2. Secure money from student government activity fees.

H. Affiliate with SASMT

1. A channel for the exchange of ideas on the national level.

FORMING A STATE ORGANIZATION

I. Prerequisites:

A. Interest and a small nucleus of students

B. Time and patience

C. Liaison with the state organization

II. Initial Organizational Steps:

A. Compile lists of:

1. Schools of Medical Technology
2. Colleges and college coordinators
3. Names and addresses of students

B. Plan a pre-organizational program. (Should be jointly planned by students and the state professional organization.)

C. Compile a list of possible pro tem officers from attendees

D. Hold a special meeting in order to:

1. Elect pro tem officers, Bylaws committee, program committee, etc.
2. Discuss objectives, etc.

III. First regular meeting:

A. Election of nominating committee

B. Election of regular officers

IV. Incidentals needed by the organization:
   A. Finances to cover mailing
   B. Access to mimeograph machine

V. Obtaining state charter:
   Contact president of state constituent society of ASMT for assistance and information about state bylaws.

Alpha Delta Theta

Two organizations for student medical technologists, one founded at Marquette University and the other at the University of Minnesota, joined together in 1944 to form Alpha Delta Theta. Its objectives are:

1. To promote social and intellectual fellowship among its members, and
2. To raise the prestige of medical technologists by inspiring its members to greater group and individual effort.

Eligibility is based on high scholastic rank, high moral ideals, and an active enthusiasm for medical technology. Its members must have received or be working toward a degree through an approved curriculum in an accredited college. Membership is limited to women.[10]

INDEPENDENT REGISTRIES

A number of independent registries have been established in laboratory specialties. The listing of these is by no means complete but includes representative groups that may be of particular interest to medical technologists.

National Certification Agency for Medical Laboratory Personnel

The National Certification Agency for Medical Laboratory Personnel (NCAMLP) was incorporated in 1977 by a group of technologists who wanted to correct what they perceived as long-identified deficiencies in the system of certifying personnel.[11]

NCAMLP was established with the announced intention to provide:

1. An autonomous credentialing agency free of pressure from a parent group or outside organization.*
2. A vehicle for cooperation among professional organizations and for standardizing the innumerable criteria for certification of personnel;
3. Certifying examinations that are competency-based and criterion-referenced;
4. A mechanism for periodic recertification.

The first certification examinations to be offered by NCAMLP were administered in July, 1978. These examinations, for Clinical

---

* On January 17, 1977, the Board of Directors of the ASMT appropriated $50,000.00 for potential fund requirements of the NCAMLP.

Laboratory Scientists (CLS) and Clinical Laboratory Technicians (CLT), were stated to have been prepared with the assistance of a private testing firm.

The eligibility requirements for taking the NCAMLP competency examination for CLS are:

1. graduation from a structured educational program in the clinical laboratory sciences which culminated in a baccalaureate degree; *or*

2. completion of a baccalaureate program which includes a minimum of 36 hours, or the equivalent, in the biological and physical sciences, plus completion of a clinical laboratory program recognized by a government agency; *or*

3. completion of a baccalaureate program which includes 36 semester hours, or the equivalent in the biological and physical sciences, plus two years of clinical laboratory experience encompassing the four major disciplines of laboratory practice—hematology, chemistry, immunology, and microbiology—within the past five years; *or*

4. completion of 60 semester hours, or the equivalent, of college course work including 36 semester hours, or the equivalent, in the biological and physical sciences, plus 10 years of work experience encompassing the four major disciplines of laboratory practice—hematology, chemistry, immunology, and microbiology.

An applicant for the CLT examination offered by NCAMLP must meet one of the following criteria:

1. graduation from a structured education program that is accredited by agencies recognized by the U.S. Office of Education or the Council on Postsecondary Education;

2. possession of a certificate of military laboratory specialist: MOS92B30, NEC 8501, NEC 8506, AFSC 90450, or AFSC 90470;

3. possession of suitable credentials from a foreign country (such credentials to be evaluated individually on receipt of evaluation);

4. possession of notarized evidence of four years of work experience encompassing the major disciplines of laboratory practice—hematology, chemistry, immunology, and microbiology.

NCAMLP announced that CLT and CLS certificates would be granted to individuals who hold appropriate government licenses, and that persons who hold certifications from other agencies in appropriate laboratory fields would also be recognized.

Certification examinations for clinical laboratory specialists had not been developed by NCAMLP at the end of 1978, nor had examinations for recertification or laboratory personnel.

The emergence of NCAMLP on the laboratory credentialing scene created considerable discussion among laboratory professionals across the nation. It created even more discussion and some amount of consternation among students, who were concerned about whether they should take the ASCP Board of Registry examination, the NCAMLP examination, or both. Some students (and medical technology program officials) expressed great concern for the employment outlook for new graduates, should they decide to sit for the "wrong" exam prior to applying for their first job. Questions such as these are by no means resolved as this book goes to press, and they are likely to remain the subject of concern for a number of years.

National Registry in Clinical Chemistry

The National Registry in Clinical Chemistry is sponsored by six boards and associations of chemists and pathologists. It evaluates the education and competency of clinical laboratory specialists in chemistry who voluntarily present their credentials to the Registry. Certification is granted at two levels: Clinical Chemistry Technologist and Clinical Chemist. The Clinical Chemistry Technologist level exists principally for applicants with recent bachelor's or master's degrees in chemistry, or for those with academic degrees in other disciplines who regularly perform clinical chemistry determinations. The level of Clinical Chemist is designed for more experienced graduates who have majored in chemical science and who are active in the field of clinical chemistry. All applicants must take an examination designed to test their practical knowledge of the fundamentals of clinical chemistry.

National Registry of Microbiologists

The National Registry of Microbiologists, which is sponsored by the American Academy of Microbiology, examines the training and competence of microbiologists at the postbaccalaureate level. Applicants must take an examination in general microbiology and in two areas of specialization. The latter may be selected from (1) agricultural and industrial microbiology, (2) foods, dairy, and sanitation microbiology, (3) pathogenic bacteriology, (4) immunology and serology, (5) virology, (6) mycology, and (7) parasitology.

Registry of Specialists in Public Health and Medical Laboratory Microbiology

Also established by the American Academy of Microbiology, the Registry of Specialists in Public Health and Medical Laboratory Microbiology is intended to identify personnel who have qualifications commensurate with supervisory standards required by Medicare for independent laboratories and interstate laboratories licensed under the Clinical Laboratory Improvement Act of 1976. The Specialist category is less broad than the Microbiologist category (page 105).

American Board of Clinical Chemistry

The American Board of Clinical Chemistry is an independent incorporated organization whose functions are:

1. Establishment and enhancement of standards of competence in clinical and toxicological chemistry and
2. Certification of qualified specialists.

Certification is based on a candidate's professional record, education, experience, and the results of an examination. Those certified by the Board are called diplomates.

INTERDISCIPLINARY ASSOCIATIONS

The American Society of Allied Health Professions was founded in 1967 as the Association of Schools of Allied Health Professions. The name was changed in 1973 to reflect the changes in membership and in the organization of the Society. It is composed of three councils: the Council of Educational Institutions, the Council of Professional Organizations, and the Council of Individual Members. The Board of Directors is composed of elected representatives from each of the three councils plus five officers.

Its purposes are:

1. To provide leadership in education for schools, colleges, divisions, and departments of allied health professions and to serve as their representative and spokesman.
2. To provide a medium for cooperation and communication among schools, colleges, divisions, and departments of allied health professions.
3. To promote the development of new allied health programs.
4. To encourage research and study of the development and evaluation of new needs and approaches in allied health fields.
5. To provide liaison with other health organizations, professional groups, and educational and governmental institutions.

REFERENCES

1. American Society of Clinical Pathologists: Newsletter for Members *I* (1): 1970.
2. Brown, Roma: Letter to ASMT Members and Non-Member Registrants. October 10, 1969.
3. American Society for Medical Technology: *ASMT STORY*, March 1974 printing.

4. Bylaws and Society Regulations of the American Society for Medical Technology, revised June 1973.

5. News Release, May 16, 1969, American Society of Medical Technologists.

6. American Medical Technologists: A.M.T. Application for Registration as an M.T.; Ridge Park, Ill. 1978 revision.

7. American Medical Technologists: A.M.T. Application for Registration as an M.L.T.; Park Ridge, Ill. 1978 revision.

8. ISCLT Recruitment Brochure, 1978.

9. Handout sheet, 1970 annual convention, American Society of Medical Technologists.

10. *Baird's Manual of American College Fraternities*. 18th ed. Menasha, Wisconsin, George Banta Co., 1968.

11. Cicarelli, S. M.: Introducing: A new certifying agency for the laboratory field. MLO, April, 1978.

SUGGESTED READINGS

Short descriptions of many organizations pertaining to the laboratory fields will be found in the annual issue of Lab World called Labstracts, usually appearing in February. Information regarding either Labstracts or Lab World may be obtained from North American Publishing Company, 401 N. Broad St., Philadelphia, Pa. 19108.

10

Supportive Personnel and Other Certifications

As laboratory medicine becomes more complicated and diverse, there is a concomitant need for greater numbers of workers. Medical technologists can make more effective and efficient use of their academic background and clinical training by delegating some of the simpler tasks to workers who have less training. These supportive personnel are presently titled laboratory assistants (LA) and medical laboratory technicians (MLT). One criterion other than training by which they can be differentiated is the degree of independent judgment they can be expected to exercise. Since these workers lack the scientific background and the depth of training required to exercise a high degree of judgment, it is necessary that they be supervised by more highly trained personnel, in this case, the medical technologist.

SUPPORTIVE PERSONNEL

It is most important that the student in medical technology understands the relationships between the medical technologist and the supportive personnel, and the basic training requirements for each category.

When the proposal for the Registry was made to the American Society of Clinical Pathologists, it suggested three classes of laboratory workers: medical technologists, laboratory technicians, and laboratory assistants. The committee, however, did not recommend the acceptance of the latter. With the low minimum standards outlined for laboratory technicians such proliferation would have been unwise and no doubt this was the argument that was effectively used to eliminate the category of laboratory assistants.

The increase in the laboratory work load immediately after World War II emphasized the need for another category of workers. The name *laboratory assistant* was proposed. Although resistance to the new category was evident in the reluctance of both the Registry and the ASMT to accept it, nevertheless it was adopted as a special certification in 1947. Dr. Montgomery[1] describes the experiment as follows: "It was almost a complete fiasco, because only a handful applied for the examination. On study of their qualifications and subsequent history most of them were found to be lacking in some element of education or training that made it impossible for them to take the examination for regular medical technologist certification. Suffice it to say, this certification 'died on the vine'." Only 100 were certified as laboratory assistants during the period this category existed.

In 1960 the Board of Directors of the American Society for Medical Technology appointed a committee to study the desirability of a program for training subprofessional workers. Their report to the 1962 convention recommended such a program. The Board of Certified Laboratory Assistants was organized in 1963 with members from both ASCP and ASMT. The board operated independently from the Board of Schools.

The standards of training for laboratory assistants are similar in many respects to those required for the approved medical technology program. There must be adequate physical space, library facilities, a competent teaching staff, and at least one instructor for every two students. The latter applies to clinical facilities only.

Some programs are set up in conjunction with a vocational school or a community college. (These programs now in community colleges are expected to be dropped in favor of the medical laboratory technician program.) Instruction in theory is given in the academic institution, and the clinical experiences are obtained at a cooperating medical facility. The period of training must be at least 12 months. Although a school of medical technology and one for laboratory assistants can be conducted by the same institution, there must be complete physical separation of instruction.

The original Code of Ethics, which was dropped at the same time the code for technologists was dropped by the Registry, included the paragraph that appears on the next page.

> Recognizing the limitations of my duties, I shall work at all times under the supervision of a qualified doctor of medicine and/or a medical technologist who is registered by the American Society of Clinical Pathologists and who abides by the Code of Ethics of that profession.

The code is included here to give historical perspective to the development of this category of workers.

The American Society of Clinical Pathologists announced in 1968 that another category of laboratory workers to be called *medical laboratory technician* was to be created. The ASMT did not endorse this move for several reasons. The general public was considered unable to distinguish between laboratory assistants and medical technologists, and it was felt that the addition of still another category would simply compound the confusion. The ASMT was in favor, however, of accepting the new category, provided the LA classification was eliminated.

The American Society of Clinical Pathologists proceeded without consultation with medical technologists, and the category of medical laboratory technician was established.

The first examination for medical laboratory technicians was given by the Registry in November, 1969. Twenty-six men and women successfully passed the examination and received certificates. Before the establishment of this category, several community colleges had set up medical laboratory technician programs, despite the fact that the only certification open to their graduates was that of laboratory assistant.

One of the problems presented by the existence of three levels of laboratory workers has been a lack of definition and general understanding of duties and responsibilities. In 1973 the ASMT approved position papers which define the various levels. These position papers were approved by democratic action of the society. They have been approved by NAACLS and the Board of Registry and have been endorsed by ASCP. The position papers are reproduced with the permission of the American Society for Medical Technology.

Laboratory Assistant (LA)

The following capabilities are expected of the LA at career entry:

> *Performing analyses:* He shall be able to perform the repetitive uncomplicated procedures, use common instruments and recognize obvious problems. These involve single-step processes where discrimination is clear, errors are few and easily corrected, and results or procedures can be confirmed with a reference test or source within the working area. Maximum proficiency in following a set of prescribed instructions, strategies and criteria is expected.

Solving problems: Decisions are made with the aid of simply stated, predetermined criteria or strategies.

Systems control, organization and communication: The ability to report work performed fully and clearly is expected.

Supervision and management: He shall be responsible for his own work as assigned by the supervisor.

Teaching others: Teaching responsibilities include only the demonstration of the performance of routine procedures when assigned to do so by his supervisor or an educational director.

Continuing education: This person shall participate in some form of continuing education or in-service program.

It is expected that this person will function at a maximum degree of effectiveness in professional attitudes, patient relations, and integrity. The group of workers represented by this level has had a structured program of clinical training.

Medical Laboratory Technicians (MLT)

In addition to the capabilities of a LA, the MLT is expected to have these capabilities.

Performing analyses: He shall be able to perform all of the repetitive tests in an up-to-date medical laboratory. This includes discrimination between closely similar items and correction of errors by use of pre-set strategies. This requires a knowledge of specific techniques and instruments and the ability to recognize factors which directly affect procedures and results. For confirmation of results, knowledge of more than one test within each specialty area is expected. He shall be able to use and monitor quality control programs within predetermined parameters. He shall be able to perform simple maintenance of instruments.

Solving problems: It is expected that he shall be able to follow prescribed strategies to recognize a problem, to identify direct causes (technical or instrumental) and to make simple corrections. It is expected that predetermined criteria will be available which anticipate problems and specify alternatives from which decisions may be made. At points where no pre-set criteria for decision making are available, the MLT would be expected to consult the supervisor.

Systems control, organization and communication: He shall be able to log in specimens, keep accurate records, prepare reports, and transmit reports clearly and completely.

Supervision and management: He shall be responsible for his work and capable of assuming responsibility for the work of the person in a direct, supportive position if asked to do so by his supervisor. Usually, he supervises only one or two people. He is also expected to have the ability to evaluate subordinates and students when asked to do so by his supervisor.

Teaching others: Teaching responsibilities include only the demonstration of the performance of routine procedures when assigned to do so by his supervisor or an educational director.

Continuing education: Active participation in continuing education and in-service programs is expected.

It is expected that this person will function at a maximum degree of effectiveness

111

in professional attitudes, patient relations and integrity. The group of workers representing this level of expectancies have associate degrees which include courses in the professional field as well as clinical experience.

Medical Technologists (MT)

The MT has completed an academic program with courses in the professional field, as well as clinical experience, and has earned a bachelor's degree. These additional capabilities are expected of him at the beginning of his career.

Performing analyses: He shall be able to perform complex analyses which require a complex network of steps and variables, fine-line discrimination of several items, correction of a variety of errors, and use and maintenance of complicated instruments. This necessitates an in depth knowledge of techniques, principles and instruments and their interrelationships. In order to confirm results he must be able to recognize interdependency of tests and must have knowledge of physiological conditions affecting test results. Since many analyses performed at this level have no means of confirmation, the MT is expected to have the capability and resourcefulness which permits him to assume the responsibility and accountability for accurate results. An expectation of major importance is the ability to establish and monitor quality control programs. He is expected also to be able to modify or design procedures.

Solving problems: He is expected to be able to recognize a problem, identify the cause (technical, instrumental or physiological), synthesize alternatives and determine solutions. This ability should extend to implementing the solution where appropriate. He shall be able to handle problems which are anticipated as well as those which are unexpected. This level of worker is expected to be able to make decisions based on a resource of information, facts, and concepts as well as foresight, judgment, and sensitivity to contributing factors. He should be able to prepare criteria and strategies which would assist subordinates in solving anticipated problems or guiding them in making routine decisions (i.e., use of quality control).

Systems control, organization and communication: Expected competencies in this area will range from keeping simple records (logging of specimens, recording results, etc.) to preparing budgets and schedules. It may further involve knowledge and understanding of the complicated operations associated with computerization of records. He must have communication skills in translating ideas and facts to a variety of persons both within and beyond the limits of the laboratory.

Supervision and management: He is expected to be responsible for his own work and decisions; to be aware of basic management skills; to be capable of supervising others and to be accountable for all work performed in his area of supervision. These responsibilities will require the basic evaluation of procedures, equipment, and people (peers, students, subordinates) and will require a knowledge of facts, concepts, skills in techniques and instruments, as well as knowledge of personnel relations and group functions.

Teaching others: Teaching responsibilities may vary from simply assisting someone else and/or bench teaching to designing, implementing and evaluating a teaching-learning experience through informal and formal programs (undergraduate, graduate and continued education).

Continuing education: It is expected that this level of worker will actively participate in continuing education and in-service programs, especially recognizing his responsibility to continue learning in areas of need, such as educational methodology, managerial skills, evaluation techniques and future planning.

It is expected that this person will function at a maximum degree of effectiveness in professional attitudes, patient relations and integrity.

OTHER CERTIFICATIONS OFFERED BY THE ASCP BOARD OF REGISTRY

Three basic types of certification are offered by the Registry: general, categorical, and specialist. The first includes medical technologists, laboratory assistants, and medical laboratory technicians.

Categorical Certifications

BLOOD BANKING. The candidate must be certified as a medical technologist and must have completed advanced training in blood banking in a blood bank approved by the American Association of Blood Banks (AABB). He must take both a written and a practical examination given by the Registry in cooperation with the AABB. The title of the person completing the training and the examinations is SBB(ASCP).

CHEMISTRY. The candidate must have a baccalaureate degree with a major in chemistry, plus one year of experience in chemistry in an acceptable laboratory. An examination is given, and the title is C(ASCP).

MICROBIOLOGY. The baccalaureate degree with a major in microbiology plus one year of experience in an acceptable laboratory are required for certification in microbiology. The title is M(ASCP).

HEMATOLOGY. Certification in medical technology plus one year of satisfactory hematology experience in an acceptable laboratory, or a baccalaureate degree in biological sciences or chemistry plus two years of satisfactory hematology experience in an acceptable laboratory are requirements for certification in hematology. A baccalaureate degree with a combination of 30 semester hours of chemistry and biology can be used to meet the academic requirements. The title is H(ASCP).

NUCLEAR MEDICAL TECHNOLOGY. The candidate must have certification in medical technology plus one year of satisfactory experience in an acceptable clinical radioisotope laboratory, or a baccalaureate degree in biological science, physical science, or chemistry, plus two years of satisfactory experience in an acceptable clinical radioisotope laboratory. The title is NM(ASCP).

HISTOLOGIC TECHNICIAN. Certification in histologic technique has been available since 1947. Growth of accredited training programs has been slow, and in 1976, only twenty-six approved programs were operating. The only admission requirement is graduation from high school. The training program is one year in length unless it is an integral part of a community college program culminating in an Associate Degree, in which case at least six months of the program must be devoted to clinical training. Successful passing of a written examination entitles the person to a certificate and the privilege of using HT(ASCP) after his name.

CYTOTECHNOLOGY. Prior to acceptance, the candidate must have two years of college credits (60 semester hours) including 12 hours of science. The course consists of at least twelve months of training in an approved school of cytotechnology. There are a few cytotechnology educational programs (such as the one at the Louisiana State University Medical Center) which require three years of college preparation prior to admission, and which culminate in the baccalaureate degree. Practical and written examinations are required for certification.

This certification has proved popular because of financial support provided for the year of training by the American Cancer Society. In some areas the support has been withdrawn because of lack of positions.

There is a shortage of cytotechnologists in most areas. The work is tedious to some, but the monetary compensation is excellent. In a large department there is always a possibility for advancement to supervisor or teaching supervisor if the hospital has a school. The work should be of particular interest to the physically handicapped, especially to those who have difficulty standing.

Specialist Certifications

There are specialist certifications available in hematology, microbiology, chemistry, and cytotechnology. The pretechnical requirements are a master's degree or doctorate in the specialty, plus three years of experience in the specialty in an acceptable laboratory. If the applicant already holds a medical technologist's certificate, there is a requirement of five years of "appropriate experience in a recognized laboratory" that has "a large volume and wide variety of procedures in the special fields." The titles are SH(ASCP); SM(ASCP); SC(ASCP); and SCT(ASCP).

There are exceptions in academic preparation and training as prerequisites for most of these certifications. Up-to-date information can always be obtained from the Registry of Medical Technologists, American Society of Clinical Pathologists.

In the years from 1969 to 1977 the specialty categories showed a popularity not previously experienced (Table 10-1). This popularity may be due to an increased need for some type of certification. It may also indicate a trend from the generalist laboratory worker to the specialist.

TABLE 10-1. ASCP Specialist Certifications

Specialty	Year Certification Began	Certificates Granted	
		through 1969	through 1977
Microbiology	1952	36	378
Chemistry	1954	19	296
Hematology	1968	8	309

REFERENCES

1. Montgomery, Lall G.: A short history of the Registry of Medical Technologists of the American Society of Clinical Pathologists. Amer. J. Clin. Path. 53:433-46, 1970.

2. Registry of Medical Technologists of the American Society of Clinical Pathologists, June, 1970. Brochure.

3. ASMT News, December, 1969.

4. Summary of the minutes, House of Delegates, 1970 Convention, ASMT News, August, 1970.

    Information regarding the various kinds of certification has been obtained from the brochure issued by the Registry of Medical Technologists of the American Society of Clinical Pathologists, June, 1970.

11

Personnel Policies

Hospitals have been much slower than industry in adopting clearly defined personnel policies in areas other than salaries, vacations, sick leave, and meals. Because every student is a potential working medical technologist and because the world of work involves personnel policies, it is of interest and importance to students to consider these policies.

Almost every medical technologist who accepts a position in a hospital laboratory will become involved at some time in discussion of fringe benefits, either because the benefits available are not as extensive as desired or because they are few or nonexistent. Often the technologists have no clear-cut plan of action to attempt to increase benefits, and their arguments are ineffective.

The Personnel Relations and Services Committee of the American Society of Medical Technologists submitted a list of recommended minimum personnel policies to the 1972 convention of ASMT. It was approved by the Board of Directors and the House of Delegates.[1]

ASMT RECOMMENDED MINIMUM PERSONNEL POLICIES
1972

1. *Hours of work:* Hours of each day shall be consecutive. Whenever possible five consecutive days totaling forty hours shall be scheduled. Hours of work on all work schedules shall comply with State and Federal regulations.

116

2. *Overtime:* Overtime shall consist of time worked at the request of the employer in excess of forty hours per week or eight hours per day during an eighty hour pay period. Overtime shall be compensated for at the rate of time and one-half.

3. *Shift differential:* Based upon the traditional three shifts per day, there shall be a shift differential of no less than five per cent for the evening shift and ten per cent for the night shift.

4. *Call time:* On Call: If not called out, the employee shall receive half-time pay for all time spent on call. Call Back: If called back, the employee is to receive time and one-half pay on a portal to portal basis for the time worked with a guarantee of one hour minimum pay for any one call.

5. *Seniority:* In a reduction of personnel, seniority shall not be the sole factor but shall be taken into consideration.

6. *Vacations:* Vacations with pay shall be allowed and shall begin with the date of employment, but not be taken in any part until the employee has worked at least six months. Cumulative vacation shall be paid if due, even though the employee terminates employment at the end of the year. After six months, vacation shall be due him on a prorated basis depending on the length of service.
   a. one to two years employment—ten working days.
   b. three to ten years employment—fifteen working days.
   c. over ten years employment—twenty working days.

7. *Sick leave:* One day of sick leave per month shall be allowed commencing with the completion of the first month employment. Sick leave shall be allowed to accumulate to a minimum of forty-five days.

8. *Holidays:* A minimum of eight paid holidays per year shall be recognized. An employee shall be eligible for holiday pay commencing with the completion of his first month of employment.

9. *Maternity leave:* After one year of employment, a minimum of three months maternity leave without pay may be granted without affecting the employee's seniority status.

10. *Pension plan:* After two years of employment, all employees shall be eligible for a pension plan in addition to Social Security.

11. *Educational leave:* After three years of employment, one year of educational leave without pay shall be granted without affecting the employee's seniority status.

12. *Continuing education:* At least three days per year and all expenses shall be allowed by the employer to attend seminars, workshops, short courses or scientific sessions offered by their professional societies at local, state and national meetings and conventions. The employer should encourage employees to continue their education through membership and participation in the affairs of their professional societies.

13. *Medical benefits:* Employees shall be eligible for Blue Cross-Blue Shield (or its equivalent), major medical, and disability insurance paid for by the employer. Employees shall also have the benefit of an employee health program and use of the hospital's ancillary service at reduced rates or at no charge.

14. *Life insurance:* All employees shall be eligible for employer-paid life insurance.

15. *Rest periods:* A fifteen minute break shall be granted during each four hours of work scheduled.

16. *Meals:* When the length of the meal break restricts the employee to the premises, meals shall be provided at a reduced rate in the employee's cafeteria.

17. *Job description:* Each employee shall be provided with a written copy of his job description.

18. *Employee evaluation:* Each employee shall be evaluated annually for economic advancement and semi-annually for performance promotion. A method which contrasts an employee's performance against pre-established objectives and against his own prior performance is recommended.

19. *Grievance procedures:* Employees shall be allowed to express complaints and grievances by established procedures similar to those recommended by the American Hospital Association.

20. *Severance pay:* No employee shall be discharged without at least two weeks notice, or severance pay in lieu of such notice, nor shall he leave without giving similar notice to his employer.

It should be remembered that this list of recommended policies is exactly what its name implies. It is a list of recommendations and not a list of demands. It should also be noted that the laboratory personnel should not expect preferential treatment from the hospital administration. If the hospital does not have a pension plan, the medical technologists cannot expect that such a plan will be set up for their particular benefit. Such circumstances call for a combined effort of all hospital employees to change administrative policies.

The question of possible recourse arises if negotiations for salary increases and/or fringe benefits fail. Every technologist looking for a position has the opportunity and the obligation to learn what benefits a particular position offers. If he does not approve the personnel policies, he can investigate other positions, provided, of course, he is not restricted to a geographic area by other considerations. Once he has accepted a position and become involved in discussions of benefits, he soon finds there is no one solution that fits every situation. In some situations the solution is dictated by the type of agreement between the hospital and the pathologist. In others, the only recourse may appear to be acceptance of the present situation or transfer to another position.

Every technologist should be aware of the ASMT Policy on Economic Negotiations.[2] It reads: "The philosophy of the American Society for Medical Technology requires that the profession place patient care above self-interest. Individual members are dedicated to uphold rigid standards of duty and performance. Patient care is jeopardized by working conditions which fail to provide proper training and adequately compensated laboratory professionals. If collective bargaining becomes necessary, negotiation by ASMT and its constituent societies is consistent with the Society's responsibility to the public."

Vertical Mobility

Vertical mobility, or the movement upwards within a profession or an occupation, can be illustrated by the man who starts his working career as a bag boy in a grocery store and concludes it as chairman of the board of directors of a food chain without completing any further academic study. Such mobility does not exist in medical technology. It is not possible to start as a glass washer in the laboratory and then to become a pathologist without any intervening academic work. Nor would such mobility be desirable from the standpoint of patient care. However, there are a number of areas in which some mobility should be possible.

Medical technology, along with many other professions, is confronted with the problem of providing for mobility within the present requirements of academic background and technical training. The American Society for Medical Technology is actively investigating the possibility of equivalency and competency testing, either for credit or for advanced placement. At the present time there is no provision for reducing the required training period for those who have had some type of training at a level below the baccalaureate. For example, a person who has completed the requirements for the Medical Laboratory Technician certificate cannot become a certified medical technologist without completing one full year of laboratory training, even though he now meets the academic prerequisites. Neither can a working technician who has had on-the-job training and years of experience become a certified technologist without completing the academic prerequisites.

The ASMT realizes the need for identification of areas where equivalency testing can be used and has appointed a committee to work on possible solutions. This committee is also working with the College Entrance Examination Board (CEEB) to develop examinations that will adequately test a candidate in areas related to the academic preparation for training.

The 1970 House of Delegates of ASMT directed that the Society (1) explore the job ladder concept as it relates to the medical laboratory, (2) develop such criteria for vertical mobility as may be realistic, desirable, and in the interest of public health and medical technology, and (3) develop a policy statement on vertical mobility.[3]

From a practical viewpoint it will be necessary to correlate the work of the committee on equivalency with that of any committee or committees appointed to carry out the mandate of the convention. If all the work is assigned to the committee on equivalency, it will be a task of gigantic proportions indeed. It is almost inevitable that progress in these areas will be slow, for the job ladder concept, although highly desirable, is complicated and multifaceted.

Medical Technology—A Perspective

Medical technology is a profession that offers challenges, opportunities, and great personal satisfactions. It offers the challenges of the new and the untried, the methods and procedures that are still just shadowy possibilities. It offers the challenge that one of these new methods may be the means of confirming the diagnosis or the cause of a disease about which little is now known. It offers opportunities to serve mankind, to advance in one's chosen profession, to contribute to research, and to increase the status and prestige of the profession. It offers the satisfaction of a meaningful contribution to total patient care. It does not promise that every day will be filled with drama and suspense, although there will be moments when a life is literally in the hands of a medical technologist. There will be the pleasure of teaching a student, of watching him develop a sense of professionalism. There will be the quiet satisfaction in the knowledge of a task well done. This is the profession of medical technology.

REFERENCES

1. Personnel Relations and Service Committee, ASMT: Report to the 1972 convention.

2. Summary of the minutes, House of Delegates, 1969 convention. ASMT News, August, 1969.

3. Summary of the minutes, House of Delegates, 1970 convention. ASMT News, August, 1970.

SUGGESTED READINGS

1. News and views. Lab. World *21*:770-772, 1970.

2. Peery, Thomas M.: Laboratory medicine: Careers and challenges. Lab. Med. *1*:32-35, 1970.

APPENDIX

Addresses of Professional Organizations and Credentialing Agencies

Accrediting Bureau of Health Education Schools
Oak Manor Office, 29089 U.S. 20 West
Elkhart, Indiana 46514

American Society of Clinical Pathologists
2100 W. Harrison St., Chicago, Ill. 60612

College of American Pathologists
230 N. Michigan Ave., Chicago, Ill. 60601

American Society for Medical Technology
5555 W. Loop S., Suite 200, Bellaire, Texas 77401

American Society for Microbiology
1913 I St. N.W., Washington, D.C. 20006

American Society of Parasitologists
University of Texas Southwestern Medical School
5323 Harry Hines Blvd., Dallas, Texas 75235

American Medical Technologists
710 Higgins Rd., Park Ridge, Ill. 60068

International Association of Medical Laboratory Technologists
% Mr. Guy Pascoe, Executive Director
No. 1 Drayton Gardens, Winchmore Hill, London, England N21-2NE

International Society for Clinical Laboratory Technology
Suite 918, 818 Olive Street, St. Louis, Mo. 63101

Board of Registry
American Society of Clinical Pathologists
P.O. Box 4872
Chicago, Illinois 60680

National Accrediting Agency for Clinical Laboratory Sciences
Suite 1512, 222 S. Riverside Plaza
Chicago, Illinois 60606

National Certification Agency for Medical Laboratory Personnel
P.O. Box 2621
Amherst, New York 14226

American Board of Bioanalysis
Suite 918
818 Olive St.
St. Louis, Mo. 63101

American Board of Clinical Chemistry
1155 16th St., N.W.
Washington, D.C. 20036

American Board of Medical Microbiology
% American Society for Microbiology
1913 Eye St., N.W.
Washington, D.C. 20006

American Registry of Radiologic Technologists
645 N. Michigan Ave.
Chicago, Ill. 60612

National Registry in Clinical Chemistry
1155 16th St., N.W.
Washington, D.C. 20036

National Registry of Microbiologists
% American Society for Microbiology (see above)

Nuclear Medicine Technology Board
475 Park Avenue South, 15th Floor
New York, N.Y. 10016

American Academy of Cytology
George L. Wied, M.D.
5841 Maryland Ave.
Chicago, Ill. 60637

GLOSSARY

Employment Categories as Defined in ASMT's 1974 Salary Survey

Administrative technologist—Plans, organizes, and delineates duties and responsibilities of personnel under direction of the director of laboratories. Duties 100% in administration.

Chief technologist—Is responsible to either the laboratory director or the administrative technologist. May spend as much as 50% of his/her time in administration. Plans, organizes, and supervises the technical activities of the laboratory.

Supervisor—May be interchangeable with chief technologist. Supervises one or more departments of the clinical laboratory.

Senior technologist or section head—Primary responsibility is co-ordination and supervision of a particular department or section.

Staff technologist—Performs in one or more areas of the clinical laboratory. Primary duty does not include supervision.

Laboratory technician—Performs laboratory procedures under supervision of staff technologist or supervisor. Results are reviewed and reported by supervising technologist.

Laboratory assistant—Performs under supervision mechanical and routine procedures that require minimum judgment.

Histologic technologist—One who prepares tissues and body materials for the study of cellular and structural characteristics by the pathologist.

Microscopy—Examination of minute objects by means of a microscope. In the clinical laboratory the term is usually applied to the area in which urinalyses are done.

Multiphasic screening—Screening of the patient by means of 20 to 40 bio-chemical and physiological determinations, the process being made possible by automation. Large segments of population could be tested at a cost of $15 to $30 per person. The information would be coded and stored in data banks. Since most of those tested would be considered to be well, early identification of hitherto unknown patterns of biochemical changes in illness could be accomplished. The role of the laboratory would change from its present role in the diagnosis and treatment of diseases to providing information needed for the maintenance of health.

Mycology—Study of the fungi, yeasts, and molds of medical importance.

Nuclear medicine—That specialty of medicine in which radioactive materials are utilized for diagnostic and therapeutic purposes.

Phlebotomist—One who obtains a sample of blood by insertion of a needle into a blood vessel.

Physiologic chemistry—Study of chemical changes in living organisms. Biochemistry. Most determinations in the clinical laboratory are carried out on specimens of blood.

Quality control—A program to control accuracy and precision of laboratory results. Although it can be applied to any department, its most common use is in chemistry. The following description is simplified considerably. Controls of known

123

value are analyzed at the same time as the patient unknowns. The mean and standard deviation of the unknowns are calculated and the deviations from the mean are plotted. If the procedure is in good control 95 percent of the determinations should fall within ± 2 standard deviations of the known control.

Serology—Literally the study of serum. The most common test in serology is one for the diagnosis of syphilis.

Toxicology—Detection of poisons in blood, feces, urine, stomach contents, or tissues.

Virology—Study of viruses, the smallest microorganisms known.

Index

Page numbers followed by t refer to tables; page numbers followed by n refer to footnotes.

125